Lecture Notes in Computer Science 10124

Commenced Publication in 1973
Founding and Former Series Editors:
Gerhard Goos, Juris Hartmanis, and Jan van Leeuwen

Tommaso Mansi · Kristin McLeod
Mihaela Pop · Kawal Rhode
Maxime Sermesant · Alistair Young (Eds.)

Statistical Atlases and Computational Models of the Heart

Imaging and Modelling Challenges

7th International Workshop, STACOM 2016
Held in Conjunction with MICCAI 2016
Athens, Greece, October 17, 2016
Revised Selected Papers

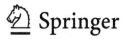 Springer

Editors

Tommaso Mansi
Siemens Medical Solutions
Medical Imaging Technologies
Princeton, NJ
USA

Kristin McLeod
Simula Research Laboratory
Oslo
Norway

Mihaela Pop
Sunnybrook Research Institute
University of Toronto
Toronto, ON
Canada

Kawal Rhode
Imaging Sciences and Biomedical
  Engineering
Rayne Institute, King's College London
London
UK

Maxime Sermesant
Inria, Asclepios Project
Sophia-Antipolis
France

Alistair Young
Department of Radiology, Faculty of
  Medical and Health Sciences
Auckland University
Auckland
New Zealand

ISSN 0302-9743   ISSN 1611-3349   (electronic)
Lecture Notes in Computer Science
ISBN 978-3-319-52717-8   ISBN 978-3-319-52718-5   (eBook)
DOI 10.1007/978-3-319-52718-5

Library of Congress Control Number: 2016963657

LNCS Sublibrary: SL6 – Image Processing, Computer Vision, Pattern Recognition, and Graphics

Preface

Recently, there has been considerable progress in cardiac image analysis techniques, cardiac atlases, and computational models, which can integrate data from large-scale databases of heart shape, function, and physiology. Integrative models of cardiac function are important for understanding disease, evaluating treatment, and planning intervention. However, significant clinical translation of these tools is constrained by the lack of complete and rigorous technical and clinical validation as well as by benchmarking of the developed tools. For doing so, common and available ground-truth data capturing generic knowledge on the healthy and pathological heart are required. This knowledge can be acquired through the building of statistical models of the heart. Several efforts are now established to provide Web-accessible structural and functional atlases of the normal and pathological heart for clinical, research, and educational purposes. We believe all these approaches will only be effectively developed through collaboration across the full research scope of the imaging and modelling communities.

STACOM 2016 was held in conjunction with the MICCAI 2016 conference (Athens, Greece) and followed on from the past six editions: STACOM 2015 (Munich, Germany), STACOM 2014 (Boston, USA), STACOM 2013 (Nagoya, Japan), STACOM 2012 (Nice, France), STACOM 2011 (Toronto, Canada), and STACOM 2010 (2010, Beijing, China). Our main goal was to organize an international event to provide a forum for the discussion of the latest developments in the areas of statistical atlases and computational imaging and modelling of the heart. The topics of the workshop included: cardiac image processing, atlas construction, statistical modelling of cardiac function across different patient populations, cardiac mapping, cardiac computational physiology, model customization, image-based modelling and image-guided interventional procedures, atlas-based functional analysis, ontological schemata for data and results, integrated functional and structural analyses, as well as the pre-clinical and clinical applicability of these methods. STACOM 2016 received many submissions from around the World, with 24 excellent papers finally accepted to be presented at the workshop and to be published in an LNCS proceedings volume by Springer. Besides regular contributions on state-of–the-art cardiac image analysis techniques, atlases, and computational models that integrate data from large-scale databases of heart shape, function and physiology, computational electrophysiology, and biomechanics, additional efforts of this year's STACOM 2016 workshop included a challenge dedicated to the segmentation of left atrial wall thickness (SLAWT), described here.

Atrial wall thickness is an important parameter for biophysical electromechanical modelling of the atria and potentially important for planning ablation therapy for atrial arrhythmias. The data were sourced at St. Thomas' Hospital, King's College London, from individuals that are being treated for atrial fibrillation and from patients with normal cardiac anatomy. The ground truth was selected by consensus manual expert annotations using the STAPLE method. Several research groups had expressed interest in participating in the challenge. Three groups had their final results submitted for evaluation. A collate paper including detailed data description and the results from participating groups was written by the SLAWT organizers and is included in these proceedings. The SLAWT data will be made publicly available via the Cardiac Atlas Project. We also anticipate a joint journal publication, as has been the case with all of our previous challenges.

We hope that the results obtained by the challenge, together with all regular paper contributions, will act to accelerate progress in the important areas of heart function and structure analysis.

In addition to the papers presented, two keynote lectures were included in the program of STACOM 2016: Dr. Sophie Mavrogeni, MD, FESC (Onassis Cardiac Surgery Centre, Athens, Greece), talk title "Cardiovascular Magnetic Resonance. Current Status and Future Applications," and Prof. Dr. Dimitris Metaxas (Rutgers University, USA), talk title "Model-Based Large-Scale Cardiac Analytics."

October 2016   Kristin Mcleod
                                                                          Tommaso Mansi
                                                                            Mihaela Pop
                                                                            Kawal Rhode
                                                                       Maxime Sermesant
                                                                          Alistair Young

Organization

We would like to thank all organizers, additional reviewers, contributing authors, and sponsors for their time, effort, and financial support in making STACOM 2016 a successful event.

Chairs

Kristin Mcleod	Simula Research Laboratory, Center for Cardiological Innovation, Oslo, Norway
Tommaso Mansi	Siemens Healthcare, Medical Imaging Technologies, Princeton, NJ, USA
Mihaela Pop	Medical Biophysics, University of Toronto, Sunnybrook Research Institute, Canada
Kawal Rhode	Imaging and Biomedical Engineering, King's College London, UK
Maxime Sermesant	Inria, Asclepios Project, Sophia Antipolis, France
Alistair Young	University of Auckland, New Zealand

SLAWT Challenge: Organizing Team

SLAWT Segmentation of Left Atrial Wall Thickness: Rashed Karim, Kawal Rhode, Oleg Aslanidi, Marta Valera, Ross Morgan, Ronak Rajani, Pranav Bhagirath

http://www.doc.ic.ac.uk/~rkarim/la_lv_framework/wall/index.html

Sponsorship Liaison

Kristin Mcleod	Simula, Oslo, Norway
Mihaela Pop	Sunnybrook Research Institute, University of Toronto, Canada

Webmaster

Avan Suinesaputra	University of Auckland, New Zealand

Workshop Website

http://stacom2016.cardiacatlas.org/

OCS (Springer Conference Submission System)

Mihaela Pop   Sunnybrook Research Institute, University of Toronto,
                       Canada
Maxime Sermensat   Inria, Asclepios Project, France

Sponsors

We are extremely grateful for the industrial funding received to support the keynote speakers, best paper/presentation prizes, and the costs of the proceedings publication.

The STACOM 2016 workshop received financial support from the following **sponsors**:

SysAfib

https://www.simula.no/research/projects/sysafib-systems-medicine-diagnosis-and-stratification-atrial-fibrillation

SciMedia Ltd

http://www.scimedia.com/

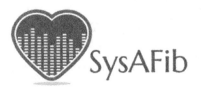

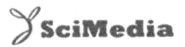

Contents

SLAWT (Segmentation of Left Atrial Wall Thickness) Challenge Papers

Regular Papers

Image-Based Real-Time Motion Gating of 3D Cardiac Ultrasound Images

Maria Panayiotou$^{(\boxtimes)}$, Devis Peressutti, Andrew P. King,
Kawal S. Rhode, and R. James Housden

Division of Imaging Sciences and Biomedical Engineering,
King's College London, London, UK
maria.panayiotou@kcl.ac.uk

Abstract. Cardiac phase determination of 3D ultrasound (US) imaging has numerous applications including intra- and inter-modality registration of US volumes, and gating of live images. We have developed a novel and potentially clinically useful real-time three-dimensional (3D) cardiac motion gating technique that facilitates and supports 3D US-guided procedures. Our proposed real-time 3D-Masked-PCA technique uses the Principal Component Analysis (PCA) statistical method in combination with other image processing operations. Unlike many previously proposed gating techniques that are either retrospective and hence cannot be applied on live data, or can only gate respiratory motion, the technique is able to extract the phase of live 3D cardiac US data. It is also robust to varying image-content; thus it does not require specific structures to be visible in the US image. We demonstrate the application of the technique for the purposes of real-time 3D cardiac gating of trans-oesophageal US used in electrophysiology (EP) and trans-catheter aortic valve implantation (TAVI) procedures. The algorithm was validated using 2 EP and 8 TAVI clinical sequences (623 frames in total), from patients who underwent left atrial ablation and aortic valve replacement, respectively. The technique successfully located all of the 69 end-systolic and end-diastolic gating points in these sequences.

Keywords: Principal component analysis · Electrophysiology · Trans-catheter aortic valve implantation · Cardiac motion gating

1 Introduction

Cardiac catheterization is a minimally invasive procedure used to diagnose and treat cardiovascular conditions. These procedures are typically performed using two-dimensional (2D) X-ray fluoroscopy which provides high-quality real-time visualization of catheters and other interventional devices. However, the cardiac anatomy itself has low contrast and can be visualized only by repeated injection of contrast agent. This makes navigation to specific targets difficult and results in long procedure times and high X-ray radiation exposure for the patient.

© Springer International Publishing AG 2017
T. Mansi et al. (Eds.): STACOM 2016, LNCS 10124, pp. 3–10, 2017.
DOI: 10.1007/978-3-319-52718-5_1

An attractive modality for imaging catheter tip placement and tissue contact to guide cardiac catheterisation procedures is ultrasound (US) [4]. US is a low-cost, non-irradiating, real-time imaging modality with good contrast for visualising anatomical structures. With the development of 2D array transducers, US has the particular advantage of providing real-time four-dimensional (4D) images of the heart. However, despite the advances in the transducer technology, gating is required to avoid motion artifacts during acquisition of large volumes. This is usually achieved by synchronising the US image acquisition with an external device, such as an electrocardiogram (ECG). Image-based gating is therefore useful as a replacement for ECG or when data is streamed live without ECG. Additionally, cardiac motion gating will be needed in any application involving intra- or inter-modality registration of US in which all images must be phase matched, e.g. automatic image-based registration of US to MRI images [3].

To date, several techniques have been developed for image-based gating in US images. Wachinger et al. [7] proposed an automatic, image-based respiratory gating method for acquiring 4D breathing data with a wobbler US probe using Laplacian eigenmaps (LE). They later developed a technique for extraction of respiratory gating navigators from US images [8]. The method was demonstrated by performing the analysis on various datasets showing different organs and sections, for both 2D and three-dimensional (3D) US data over time. Additionally, motion models have been proposed to correct for respiratory motion using US data. Peressutti et al. [6] proposed a novel framework for motion-correcting the pre-procedural information that combines a probabilistic MRI-derived affine motion model with intra-procedure real-time 3D echocardiography images in a Bayesian framework. However, these techniques are limited to only respiratory gating. An approach for retrospective end-diastolic gating of intra coronary US sequences (ICUS) using feature extraction and classification was proposed by De Winter et al. [1]. This method is computationally expensive and requires processing the whole sequence together, as some of the features are temporal. Zhu et al. [9] proposed two techniques to analyse images in the sequence and retrieve the cardiac phase from intravascular US (IVUS) images based on average image intensity and absolute difference in pixel intensity between the consecutive frames. However, the robustness of this method was not thoroughly evaluated as no precise quantified validation of this method was performed. All in all, there is no technique proposed to date that can cardiac gate live 3D US images in real-time.

A recent paper by Panayiotou et al. demonstrates that cardiac gating in X-ray using the Principal Component Analysis (PCA) statistical method is superior to Manifold Learning and phase correlation techniques [5]. In this paper a technique for automated 2D image-based retrospective cardiorespiratory motion gating in X-ray fluoroscopy images was proposed. This used the PCA statistical method in combination with other image processing operations, resulting in the Masked-PCA technique, suitable for retrospective cardiorespiratory gating. A disadvantage of this previously proposed approach and all other mentioned cardiac gating approaches is that they are retrospective and consequently, real-time application to live data is not possible. Additionally, Masked-PCA is limited to 2D cardiac gating and so is only applicable to X-ray fluoroscopic procedures. In the current paper, we significantly extend the previous approach to make it applicable to live 3D US image data. Validation of our technique is done on trans-oesophageal echo (TOE) images from electrophysiology (EP) and trans-catheter aortic valve implantation (TAVI) procedures.

2 Methods

In this section we first describe the formation of our statistical model in a training step (Sect. 2.1), which is a slight modification of the previous work on Masked-PCA [5], and then its application in a live gating step (Sect. 2.2), which is the main novel contribution of this work. The modification of our newly proposed technique in the training step was needed to make the technique applicable to 3D images, and consequently suitable for different types of US procedures. Additionally, the live gating step was introduced to make the technique suitable for real-time gating of previously unseen images, based on a statistical model formed from images during the training step. Figure 1, gives an overview of our proposed workflow.

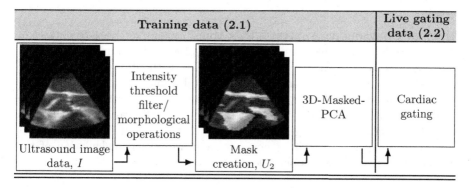

Fig. 1. Illustration of proposed workflow. The Sects. 2.1 and 2.2 refer to the corresponding section numbers in the text.

2.1 Training Step

Intensity Threshold and Morphological Operations. An intensity threshold is applied individually to all 3D images, I, in the training section of the sequence. A sensitivity analysis showed that the gating accuracy was not sensitive to the value of the threshold for values between 50–200 (150 was used here). This technique is used with the aim of identifying pixels in the images which are expected to carry useful cardiac motion information in their intensity variation over time. The thresholding was introduced as a replacement of the Frangi vesselness filter used in [5]. This is necessary because the relevant features in 3D US tend to be high-intensity planar structures rather than the 2D tubular structures seen in X-ray. Applying a threshold binarises the image. Following the method of [5], morphological opening is applied to the binarised responses to remove the noise present while preserving the shape and size of the detected structures. This is followed by the application of morphological dilation to include surrounding pixels which also vary as the structures move. We denote the result of this process by U_{1_i}, where i is the US frame number.

Mask Creation. Any pixels detected by the above image processing operations, in any frame of the training sequence, are used to create a mask, denoted by U_2 covering the movement range of any detected structures. This same mask is applied to all frames in the sequence. For each training frame, the intensities of each of the pixels in the mask were concatenated into a single column vector $\mathbf{s}_i$. Hence the data generated by this process consisted of:

$$\mathbf{s}_i = (I_{i,1}, I_{i,2}, \ldots I_{i,J})^T, 1 \leq i \leq N \tag{1}$$

where $I_{i,j}$ represents the intensity of the ith image frame at the jth pixel in the mask, U_2. N is the number of frames and J is the number of pixels within the masked region. $\mathbf{s}_i$ is the ith column of matrix $\mathbf{s}$.

Principal Component Analysis. PCA transforms a multivariate dataset of possibly correlated variables into a new dataset of a smaller number of uncorrelated variables called Principal Components (PCs), without any loss of information [2]. We first compute the mean vector over all frames, $\bar{\mathbf{s}}$, and the covariance matrix, $\mathbf{S}$. The eigenvectors $\mathbf{v}_m$, $1 \leq m \leq M$ of $\mathbf{S}$ represent the PCs and the corresponding eigenvalues d_m, $1 \leq m \leq M$ represent the variance of the data along the direction of the eigenvectors. Note that although $M = J$, at most $N - 1$ of the eigenvalues will be non-zero, and an efficient calculation of the corresponding eigenvectors is possible [5].

2.2 Live Cardiac Gating Step

For live gating, the task is to gate previously unseen images, acquired in the same view as the training data, based on the statistical model formed during the training step (Sect. 2.1). The mask U_2 calculated in the training stage is applied to the unseen image I_k producing a new data vector $\mathbf{t_k}$. We then compute the scalar projection between this unseen data and each of the PC vectors:

$$P_{m,k} = (\mathbf{t}_k - \bar{\mathbf{s}})^T \cdot \mathbf{v}_m, \quad 1 \leq m \leq M \tag{2}$$

The hypothesis is that the PCA will extract cardiac modes and that $P_{m,k}$ will therefore vary with cardiac motion and can be used for gating. It was found by correlation with the gold standard results that the variation of the 1st PC was dominated by cardiac motion. The peaks of the variation plots represent end-systolic cardiac frames while the troughs represent end-diastolic cardiac frames.

$$\Omega_{end-sys} = \{i \mid P_{1,i-1} < P_{1,i} > P_{1,i+1}\} \tag{3}$$

$$\Omega_{end-dia} = \{i \mid P_{1,i-1} > P_{1,i} < P_{1,i+1}\} \tag{4}$$

where $\Omega_{end-sys}$ and $\Omega_{end-dia}$ is the set of all frame numbers that are identified as end-systole and end-diastole, respectively. The remaining PCs were not used.

3 Experiments

3.1 Data Acquisition

All patient procedures were carried out using a Philips iE33 cardiac US scanner. The US probe was a Philips X7-2t trans-esophageal probe. This study was approved by our Local Ethics Committee. In total, the technique was tested on eight different clinical TAVI sequences (592 frames) from one patient who underwent a TAVI procedure, and two different clinical EP sequences (31 frames) from an additional patient who underwent a left atrial ablation procedure for the treatment of atrial fibrillation (AF). For all sequences, the acquired data were synchronised to the heartbeat using the three-lead ECG on the scanner. The ECG signal was employed for validation purposes.

3.2 Application of the Technique to US Sequences

In all but one sequence, two heartbeats of data were acquired, beginning just before the ECG R wave. For these sequences, the technique was validated using the leave-one-out cross-validation approach. A single frame from the original sequence was used as the validation data, and the remaining frames formed the training data to build the statistical model, for each of the frames in turn. In one TAVI sequence, the recording was longer, comprising 327 frames. In this case the model was trained on the first 26 frames (approximately one heartbeat) and was tested on the remaining frames.

Validation. To validate our technique, gold standard manual gating of the cardiac cycle at end-systole and end-diastole was performed by an experienced observer, by visually detecting the opening and closing of either the mitral or the tricuspid valve, depending on which one was visible in the images. The signals obtained using the gold standard method were then compared to the signals obtained using the model-based method, for both end-systolic and end-diastolic gating. Specifically, the absolute frame difference compared to the gold standard was computed for both end-systolic and end-diastolic frames. Motion gating accuracy objectives were set based on potential clinical applications that the proposed method could tackle. These applications include intra- or inter-modality registration of US volumes. These applications will use the end-diastolic cardiac phase, where the heart is more relaxed, and it is expected that its shape will be more repeatable over several cycles. Since the heart will be relatively stationary in the end-diastolic phase for a period of about 0.3 s, the motion gating accuracy objective is set to 0.1 s. Successful gating is signified when the absolute frame difference is within this limit.

4   Results

4.1   Gold Standard Validation

Manual gating of the cardiac cycle was further validated by two additional observers who were trained to identify the end-systolic and end-diastolic frames throughout the US sequences. The average inter-observer standard deviation was computed as a proportion of the cardiac cycle, assuming 1 s per heartbeat. Results are shown in Table 1.

Table 1. Average inter observer standard deviation as a proportion of the cardiac cycle.

Average standard deviation (s) (%)				
Gating task	No. of peaks	Average variation	No. of peaks	Average variation
	TAVI		EP	
End-systolic	32	0.015	3	0
End-diastolic	30	0.009	4	0

4.2   Cardiac Motion Gating

Qualitative Validation. Figure 2a gives an illustration of the first frame of one example TAVI sequence, I_1. Figure 2b illustrates the mask, U_2, overlaid with the corresponding US image for the first frame of the same example case (Sect. 2.1). The results of the cardiac gating validation are shown in Fig. 3a for the first 150 frames for an example sequence. Our 3D-Masked-PCA technique is shown in dashed-dot black lines. The plotted vertical red and green lines correspond to the gold standard end-systolic and end-diastolic frames, respectively.

Quantitative Validation. For both end-systolic and end-diastolic cardiac gating, the absolute frame difference between our technique and the gold standard technique can be seen in the frequency distribution bar chart in Fig. 3b. All of the 35 end-systolic peaks and 34 end-diastolic troughs were located correctly within the 0.1 s objective. No false positives or negatives (i.e. extra/fewer detected peaks/troughs) over the processed sequences were found. This outcome shows that our technique is robust and accurate in cardiac motion extraction.

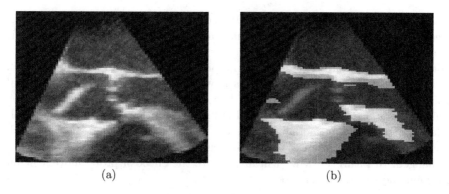

Fig. 2. (a) An US image, I_1 for one example TAVI case. (b) Mask output, U_2, overlaid with the corresponding US image of the same example case.

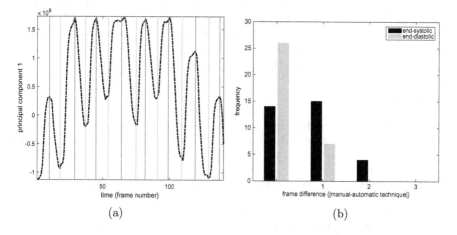

Fig. 3. (a) Graphical representation of cardiac phases obtained after applying the 3D-Masked-PCA method in dashed-dot black lines for the first 150 frames for an example US sequence. The vertical red and green lines are the gold standard identification of end-systolic and end-diastolic frames, respectively. (b) Frequency distributions of frame difference errors for end-systolic and end-diastolic US frames. (Color figure online)

Regarding our algorithm's performance on the different experiments, the execution time was between 0.0005 and 0.001 s per frame running in Matlab on Windows 7 with a 3.4 GHz Intel Core i7 CPU and 8 GB of RAM. Consequently, our technique could achieve an average frame rate of 294 f/s, which is well above that required for live US gating.

5 Discussion and Conclusions

We have presented a novel and clinically useful real-time cardiac gating technique based on PCA and have demonstrated its application for automatic cardiac gating of unseen 3D TAVI and EP TOE sequences. Unlike all previously developed motion gating techniques, the main novelty of our technique is that it is applicable to 3D images and is not retrospective. Our technique is image content independent, fully automatic, requires no prior knowledge and can operate with an average frame rate of 294 f/s. This is well above the frame rate of clinical US. Thus, real-time cardiac gating of live 3D ultrasound could potentially be achieved. The method will also be particularly useful for registration of US volumes to other imaging modalities, thereby enhancing image guidance for such interventions. A limitation of the method is the need to retrain when the view is changed. In future work we will investigate the effect of probe movement on the robustness of the technique.

Acknowledgements. We acknowledge financial support from the Department of Health via the National Institute for Health Research (NIHR) comprehensive Biomedical Research Centre award to Guy's and St Thomas' NHS Foundation Trust in partnership with King's College London and King's College Hospital NHS Foundation Trust. This work was supported by the Engineering and Physical Sciences Research Council [grant number EP/L505328/1]. We also thank Guy's and St Thomas' Department of Cardiology for providing the data used.

References

1. De Winter, S., Hamers, R., Degertekin, M., Tanabe, K., Lemos, P., Serruys, P., Roelandt, J., Bruining, N.: A novel retrospective gating method for intracoronary ultrasound images based on image properties. In: Computers in Cardiology, pp. 13–16 (2003)
2. Jolliffe, I.: Principal Component Analysis. Springer, New York (2002)
3. King, A., Rhode, K., Ma, Y., Yao, C., Jansen, C., Razavi, R., Penney, G.: Registering preprocedure volumetric images with intraprocedure 3-D ultrasound using an ultrasound imaging model. IEEE Trans. Med. Imaging **29**(3), 924–937 (2010)
4. Mackensen, G., Hegland, D., Rivera, D., Adams, D., Bahnson, T.: Real-time 3-dimensional transesophageal echocardiography during left atrial radiofrequency catheter ablation for atrial fibrillation. Circ. Cardiovasc. Imaging **1**(1), 85–86 (2008)
5. Panayiotou, M., King, A., Housden, R., Ma, Y., Cooklin, M., O'Neil, M., Gill, J., Rinaldi, C., Rhode, K.: A statistical method for retrospective cardiac and respiratory motion gating of interventional cardiac X-ray images. Med. Phys. **41**(7), 071901 (2014)
6. Peressutti, D., Penney, G., Housden, R., Kolbitsch, C., Gomez, A., Rijkhorst, E., Barratt, D., Rhode, K., King, A.: A novel bayesian respiratory motion model to estimate and resolve uncertainty in image-guided cardiac interventions. Med. Image Anal. **17**(4), 488–502 (2013)
7. Wachinger, C., Yigitsoy, M., Navab, N.: Manifold learning for image-based breathing gating with application to 4D ultrasound. In: Jiang, T., Navab, N., Pluim, J.P.W., Viergever, M.A. (eds.) MICCAI 2010. LNCS, vol. 6362, pp. 26–33. Springer, Heidelberg (2010). doi:10.1007/978-3-642-15745-5_4
8. Wachinger, C., Yigitsoy, M., Rijkhorst, E.J., Navab, N.: Manifold learning for image-based breathing gating in ultrasound and MRI. Med. Image Anal. **16**(4), 806–818 (2012)
9. Zhu, H., Oakeson, K., Friedman, M.: Retrieval of cardiac phase from IVUS sequences. In: SPIE 5035, Medical Imaging, vol. 5035, pp. 135–146 (2003)

Novel Framework to Integrate Real-Time MR-Guided EP Data with T1 Mapping-Based Computational Heart Models

Sebastian Ferguson[1], Maxime Sermesant[2], Samuel Oduneye[1,3],
Sophie Giffard-Roisin[2], Michael Truong[1,4], Labonny Biswas[1],
Nicholas Ayache[2], Graham Wright[1,3], and Mihaela Pop[1,3(✉)]

[1] Sunnybrook Research Institute, Toronto, Canada
mihaela.pop@utoronto.ca
[2] Inria - Asclepios Project, Sophia Antipolis, France
[3] Medical Biophysics, University of Toronto, Toronto, Canada
[4] Kings College London, London, UK

Abstract. Real-time MRI-guided electrophysiology (EP) interventions hold the potential to replace conventional X-ray guided procedures aimed to eliminate potentially lethal scar-related arrhythmia. Furthermore, although cardiac MR can provide excellent structural information (i.e., anatomy and scar), these catheter-based procedures have limited electrical information due to sparse electrical maps recorded from endocardial surfaces. In this paper, we propose a novel framework to augment such sparse electrical maps with 3D transmural electrical wave propagation obtained non-invasively using computer modelling. First, we performed real-time MR-guided EP studies using a preclinical pig model (i.e., in 1 healthy and 2 chronically infarcted animals). Specifically, the MR scans employed 2D T1-mapping ($1 \times 1 \times 5$ mm spatial resolution) based on a multi-contrast late enhancement method. For the EP studies we used an MR-compatible system (*Imricor*). Second, the stacks of resulting segmented images were used to build 3D heart models with various zones (i.e., healthy, scar and gray zone). Lastly, the 3D heart models were coupled with simple monodomain reaction-diffusion equations (e.g. eikonal and Aliev-Panfilov). Our simulations showed that these mathematical formalisms are advantageous due to fast computations, allowing us to predict the electrical wave propagation through dense LV meshes (e.g. >100 K elements, element size ~ 1.5 mm) in <3 min on a consumer computer. Overall, preliminary results demonstrated that the 3D MCLE-based models predicted close activation times and patterns compared to our measured EP maps, while also providing 3D transmural information and a precise location of the infarction. Future work will focus on calibrating directly (in near real-time) T1-based personalized heart models from electrical maps obtained during real-time MR-guided EP mapping procedures.

Keywords: Cardiac MRI · Modelling · Electrophysiology · Histopathology

© Springer International Publishing AG 2017
T. Mansi et al. (Eds.): STACOM 2016, LNCS 10124, pp. 11–20, 2017.
DOI: 10.1007/978-3-319-52718-5_2

1 Introduction

Ventricular tachycardia (VT), a dangerous arrhythmia, is a major cause of sudden cardiac death in patients with structural disease such as myocardial infarction (MI) [1]. In VT, an abnormal electrical wave propagates around unexcitable scars and through viable channels of reduced functionality [2]. The structural characteristics of infarcted areas are evaluated in the clinics using MR imaging, which has excellent soft tissue contrast. In addition, the changes in electrical properties due to collagenous scar development are identified in the electrophysiology (EP) lab typically under X-ray fluoroscopy, using catheter-based systems (e.g. CARTO, NOGA, Ensite). During the EP study, clinicians aim to thermally ablate the "viable channels" (i.e., the VT substrate where the foci reside). These channels are often found in the peri-infarct area and consist in a mixture of viable and non-viable myocytes. Unfortunately, the success rate of the VT ablations is currently low [1–3] due to various limitations of the EP systems (i.e., sparse electrical maps, surface data, exposure to high X-ray dose during long procedures, invasiveness of VT inducibility test, etc.).

To improve the mapping and VT ablation procedures, many centers fuse contrast-enhanced MR and EP data [4], but currently there is a clear need to further reduce: (a) the total procedure time associated with a typical MR study followed by conventional EP study, and (b) the errors between the location of scar/channels identified in MR and EP data. Thus, an attractive alternative is the use of real-time MR-guided EP systems, which employ MR-compatible catheters. Such systems have been recently implemented in several research centers in the world, with pre-/clinical feasibility studies yielding promising results [5, 6]. Notable, the MR-guided EP mapping systems do not use ionizing radiation and produce significantly lower location errors (~ 3 mm) compared to CARTO system [3].

However, despite considerable efforts and the development of complex systems, two major limitations remain the sparsity of electrical points along with the lack of transmural electrical information (since the electrical maps are recorded only from the endocardial and/or epicardial surfaces). To overcome this limitation, one can use *computational modelling* [7]. This powerful non-invasive tool can be combined with structural information extracted from cardiac MRI to build 3D anatomical models that can be used to predict the abnormal propagation of electrical impulse in the presence of non-conductive scars and to simulate the generation of VT waves looping around dense scars. We have previously used such computational tools by employing 3D MRI-based heart models (histologically validated) obtained from high-resolution *ex vivo* diffusion tensor images of explanted porcine hearts. Some of our heart models were previously personalized from surfacic EP data (i.e., maps of activation times) recorded via x-ray-guided EP systems [8].

In this work, we propose a novel preclinical framework that integrates real-time MR-guided EP data with computerized 3D models of healthy/infarcted hearts. Notable, for scar imaging we used a high-resolution T1 mapping method, recently validated using quantitative histology [10]. This gave us confidence that our 3D heart models (integrating three zones: scar, healthy tissue and channels) are anatomically accurate. We then dissected the propagation of electrical wave through the heart using fast

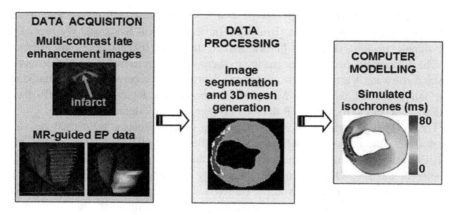

Fig. 1. Diagram of the workflow (see text for more details)

computer models. A simplified diagram of the workflow illustrating various components of the framework is included in Fig. 1.

2 Materials and Methods

2.1 Animal Preparation

In this paper we included results from three MR-EP studies performed in a pre-clinical animal model (i.e., one healthy swine and two swine with chronically infarcted hearts). All interventional procedures received approval from Sunnybrook Research Institute. The methodology of generating myocardial infarction was previously described [8]. Briefly, in this current work, the left ascending artery (LAD) was occluded by a balloon catheter for ∼90 min, followed by balloon retraction and tissue reperfusion in order to create a heterogeneous infarction that mimicked typical pathological characteristics of MI in humans.

The infarcted animals were allowed to heal for approximately 5–6 weeks prior to the MR-EP studies and to develop chronic fibrosis. By this time point, a dense collagenous scar (i.e., fibrosis) had replaced dead myocytes in the infarct core, while a mixture of viable and non-viable collagen fibrils was found in the peri-infarct. This was confirmed by a collagen-sensitive histological stain as in our previous studies [8].

2.2 Real-Time MR-Guided EP Studies and Data Processing

All MR-EP studies were performed using a 1.5 GE MR scanner. For MR imaging of the heart anatomy we used a cine SSFP sequence, while for scar detection we used our T1 mapping method based on a 2D multi-contrast late enhancement (MCLE) pulse sequence, as previously described [9]. Both types of MR images were acquired using a $1 \times 1 \times 5$ mm spatial resolution.

Our real-time MR-EP system consisted of 8.5 Fr catheters MR-compatible and a prototype EP Recording System (Bridge™, Imricor Medical Systems). We recorded MR signals, tracking data, and intracardiac electrograms (EGMs) from the catheter tip. The MR images acquired for roadmaps were sent to an in-house developed visualization software, Vurtigo (www.vurtigo.ca). Vurtigo also received real-time tracking data and converted them into MR position coordinates for fusion with EP data. Notably, MR and MR-guided EP data are co-registered (by default).

The EGM waveforms gathered from the tip of the catheters were used in conjunction with the catheter coordinates to produce endocardial activation maps. This was achieved by placing a reference catheter on the septum of the RV, and a mapping catheter in the LV. Our system simultaneously recorded the two EGMs and the coordinates of the tracking coils in the catheters. By holding the mapping catheter at one point, we were able to associate a section of the EGMs with a particular coordinate in the endocardium.

The activation time at each of these points was measured manually in Vurtigo by comparing the reference and mapping EGMs. For this, we used a caliper (Fig. 2a) that measured the delay between two peaks in the signals. Example of EGM waveforms from the tip of catheters inserted in RV (for pacing) and LV (for mapping), are shown in Fig. 2b.

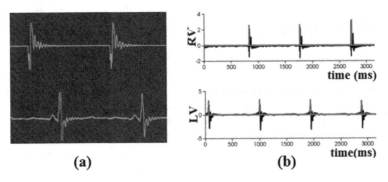

(a)   (b)

Fig. 2. Electrocardiograms recorded with the Imricor catheter and visualized in Vurtigo: (a) the caliper (in red) measures egm amplitude; and (b) example of recordings from RV and LV under pacing at 400 ms. (Color figure online)

Figure 3a shows an example of fused MR-EP data that was obtained in one infarcted pig. The endocardial contours (drawn in white) were semi-automatically detected in the prior cine SSFP images. The resulting co-registered fused MR data with the EP isochronal map is shown in Fig. 3b. Note that for the color map, early activation/depolarization times are in red and late local activation times in blue. The EGMs were further used to construct endocardial activation maps (i.e., isochrones of depolarization times). The activation maps were recorded from the endocardium of the LV, either in sinus rhythm or under pacing conditions (i.e., at 400 ms, with the pacing catheter placed in the right ventricle, RV, touching the septum).

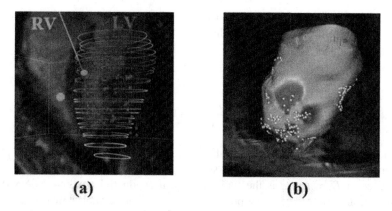

Fig. 3. Visualization of real-time MR-guided EP data in an infarcted pig heart: (a) co-registered MR-EP data; and (b) fused MR image with interpolated isochronal EP map.

For infarcted cases, the MCLE images were used to extract the steady-state and T1* maps, which were used as an input to a fuzzy-logic segmentation algorithm [9], which is a robust algorithm to cluster infarct core, peri-infarct (grey zone, GZ, where the arrhythmia substrate resides) and healthy pixels.

2.3 Mesh Generation

We generated 3D volumetric LV meshes of sufficiently high density (i.e., between 100–300 K elements, with mean element size approximately 1–1.5 mm), to capture accurately the wave propagation in the peri-infarct areas. All anatomical meshes were constructed using CGAL libraries (www.cgal.org) and Inria tools, from the stacks of segmented 2D MCLE images for infarcted pigs, and from cine SSFP images for the healthy case, respectively.

All 3D meshes integrated synthetic fiber directions generated using rule-based methods that obey analytical equations [10]. For the tissue properties corresponding to the key model parameters, we assigned a different *electrical conductivity value* per each zone (i.e., healthy tissue, slow-conductive GZ and non-conductive scar) to mimic the electrophysiological properties of chronic infarct (see below).

2.4 Computational Modelling

The 3D MCLE-based heart models were further used for simulations. Specifically, we simulated the electrical wave propagation through the heart using two fast mono-domain macroscopic formalism. We then compared the models' output (i.e., isochronal maps) and computational times (tractability) between them and also against the measured isochronal maps. Both mathematical models have a reaction-diffusion term.

The Aliev-Panfilov (A-P) model solves for the action potential (V) and recovery term (r) as described in the reaction-diffusion equations [11, 12]:

$$\frac{\partial V}{\partial t} = \nabla \cdot (D\nabla V) - kV(V - a)(V - 1) - rV \tag{1}$$

$$\frac{\partial r}{\partial t} = -(\varepsilon + \frac{\mu_1 r}{\mu_2 + V})(kV(V - a - 1) + r) \tag{2}$$

where a tunes the action potential duration and k corresponds to the recovery phase. This simplified model accounts for tissue anisotropy (i.e., fiber directions) via the diffusion tensor D, where d is the 'bulk' electrical conductivity of tissue. A reduced value of d results in a slow wave propagation, as per the relation between the speed (i.e., conduction velocity) c and d:

$$c = \sqrt{2 \cdot k \cdot d}(0.5 - a) \tag{3}$$

The Eikonal (EK) model is the fastest existing model. This fast model computes only the wave front propagation (i.e., the depolarization phase T_d of the electrical wave) based on the anisotropic Eikonal equation [13]:

$$c^2(\nabla T_d^t D \nabla T_d) = 1 \tag{4}$$

where the c is the local speed of the wave and D is the diffusion tensor as in the A-P model described above.

Note that in both computational models, we worked with the following value for speed: $c = 30$ cm/s in the GZ (which is a value reduced by 50% compared to c healthy tissue 60 cm/s). We also assigned $c = 0$ in the dense core (which is non-conductive). In both models (A-P and EK) the anisotropy ratio was set to 1:3 (to account for the anisotropic propagation of the electrical wave in transverse vs. longitudinal direction of the fiber).

For all Finite Element simulations, we used a 4,096(1x) MB machine with an Intel® Core™ i3-2310 M processor, 640 GB HD, NVIDIA® GeForce® 315 M graphic adapter.

3 Results and Discussion

Figures 4a–c show exemplary results from the construction of the 3D anatomical model from one of the infarcted hearts, with the scar in the territory of the left anterior descending artery (LAD). From the stack of 2D segmented MCLE images we obtained an interpolated 3D anatomical heart model, which integrated the three types of tissue (GZ, healthy zone and dense scar). The synthetic fibers generated using rule-based methods rotated from −70° to +70° (from endocardium to epicardium), were integrated into the 3D mesh by assigning the fiber directions at each vertex (see example in Fig. 4d).

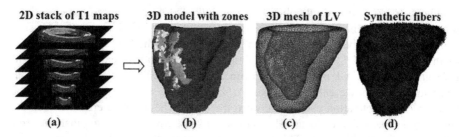

2D stack of T1 maps   **3D model with zones**   **3D mesh of LV**   **Synthetic fibers**

(a)   (b)   (c)   (d)

Fig. 4. Construction of the T1-based heart model for one infarcted heart: (a) stack of 2D segmented T1 maps; (b–c) corresponding 3D model and tetrahedral mesh (CGAL); and (d) rule-based synthetic fibers. Notable, the 3D model has three zones: healthy (dark blue), GZ (white) and dense scar (light blue) resulted from segmenting MCLE images. (Color figure online)

Figure 5 presents simulation results obtained for the healthy heart. The outputs of the both EK and A-P models were compared with the recorded endocardial EP map (which was projected onto the endocardial surface of the mesh). Overall, we observed a close correspondence between simulated and measured isochronal maps, as illustrated in Fig. 5-*top*. The A-P model yielded a slightly better match of activation pattern with and a smaller absolute error (8 ms) compared with the measured map, while the simulated isochrones by the EK model lead to a larger absolute (12 ms). Figure 5-*bottom* shows a qualitative comparison of epicardial isochrones (simulated depolarization times) using the EK and A-P models, respectively. A small difference (i.e., mean error for all vertices <5 ms) and a very good correlation coefficient (0.92) was found between the simulated isochrones predicted by A-P model vs. the EK model. Note that all quantitative comparisons were performed using in-house tools developed in Matlab.

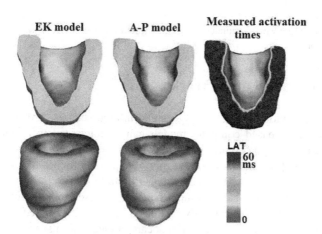

EK model   **A-P model**   **Measured activation times**

LAT
60 ms

0

Fig. 5. Comparison between simulated and measured isochrones for the healthy heart (see text for details). For the color scale, red represents the early activation time (EAT), while in blue are late activation times, LAT (ms). In the epicardial maps, EAT corresponded to the location of pacing catheter tip in the MR image. (Color figure online)

Figure 6 shows the results obtained in an infarcted heart (i.e., the same one presented in Fig. 4). The generated mesh had approximately 122 K elements. The simulations with A-P model were performed in <3 min, while the E-K simulations in 18 s (with a time-step of 1×10^{-4} s). For simplicity, we included below only the comparison between the A-P model and experimental isochrones (the latter being projected and interpolated on the endocardial mesh). Overall, there was a good correspondence between of the activation patterns between the maps. The absolute error between the simulated vs. measured endocardial values was 14 ms, which was larger than the error obtained in the healthy case. This can be explained by the fact that the endocardial measurements are sparse (e.g. <60 points), leading to small differences in the activation times within in the peri-infarct areas and adjacent zones, compared to the values computed on 3D meshes.

Overall, the 3D models give superior information compared to the surfacic EP measurements, since they allow visualization of transmural activation times and resulting activation pattern through the myocardial wall, relative to the precise position of the scar in the infarcted hearts.

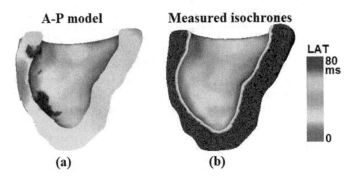

Fig. 6. Comparison between simulated (A-P model) and measured isochrones in one infarcted heart (see text for details).

4   Conclusion and Future Work

Non-invasive evaluation methods of myocardial infarct, such as cardiac MR imaging and predictive image-based computer models can be integrated to provide powerful tools for the clinicians, particularly in EP labs. Such integrative tools can be also used for surgical training [14]. In this work, we proposed a novel framework to augment the information from real-time MR image-guided EP studies with 3D simulations using high-resolution T1-mapping-based computer models. These models could supplement important information that is currently lacking during catheter-based EP procedures due to the sparse and surfacic nature of endocardial electrical maps.

Our preclinical results suggest that macroscopic theoretical models such as A-P and EK can provide very fast simulation results (in <3 min for A-P model, and <20 s for EK model, respectively) for relatively dense MR-based heart meshes, making them attractive for a rapid integration into the clinical platforms. Although these preliminary results are promising, we acknowledge that a modelling limitation was the usage of *global* parameters (i.e., same conductivity or speed within the healthy tissue of LV). Likely better predictions can be obtained if these key parameters in the A-P and EK models will be calibrated directly from measured EP maps and using the *local* 17-segment AHA model for LV.

Future work will focus on personalizing *local* model parameters per individual heart from EP data as in [15]. We envision that such refined approach will improve the model personalization, particularly in pathological hearts with structural disease. This will enable more accurate predictions of activation maps and, later, an improved outcome of MR-guided EP ablation of scar-related VT patients. Furthermore, for both rapid scar/GZ imaging and image-based model generation, we will use our newly developed high resolution 3D MCLE scan based on a reconstruction method using compressed sending [16], which will avoid cardiac motion and respiratory registration errors.

Acknowledgement. The authors are grateful for funding and support received from the CIHR, FedDev and Imricor Medical Systems.

References

1. Stevenson, W.G.: Ventricular scars and VT tachycardia. Trans. Am. Clin. Assoc. **120**, 403–412 (2009)
2. Bello, D., Fieno, D.S., Kim, R.J., et al.: Infarct morphology identifies patients with substrate for sustained ventricular tachycardia. J. Am. College Cardiol. **45**(7), 1104–1108 (2005)
3. Codreanu, A., Odille, F., et al.: Electro-anatomic characterization of post-infarct scars comparison with 3D myocardial scar reconstruction based on MRI. J. Am. Coll. Cardiol. **52**, 839–842 (2008)
4. Wijnmaalen, A., van der Geest, R., van Huls van Taxis, C., Siebelink, H., Kroft, L., Bax, J., Reiber, J., Schalij, M., et al.: Head-to-head comparison of c-e MRI and electroanatomical voltage mapping to assess post-infarct scar characteristics in patients with VT: real-time image integration and reversed registration. Eur. Heart J. **32**, 104 (2011)
5. Lardo, A.C., McVeigh, E.R., et al.: Visualization and temporal/spatial characterization of cardiac RF ablation lesions using MRI. Circulation **102**(6), 698–705 (2000)
6. Oduneye, S.O., Biswas, L., Ghate, S., Ramanan, V., Barry, J., Laish-Farkash, A., Kadmon, E., Zeidan Shwiri, T., Crystal, E., Wright, G.A.: The feasibility of endocardial propagation mapping using MR guidance in a swine model and comparison with standard electro-anatomical mapping. IEEE Trans. Med. Imaging **31**(4), 977–983 (2012)
7. Clayton, R.H., Panfilov, A.V.: A guide to modelling cardiac electrical activity in anatomically detailed ventricles. Progr. Biophys. Mol. Biol. Rev. **96**(1–3), 19–43 (2008)
8. Pop, M., Ramanan, V., Yang, F., Zhang, L., Newbigging, S., Wright, G.: High resolution 3D T1* mapping and quantitative image analysis of the gray zone in chronic fibrosis. IEEE Trans. Biomed. Eng. **61**(12), 2930–2938 (2014)

9. Pop, M., Sermesant, M., Flor, R., Pierre, C., Mansi, T., Oduneye, S., Barry, J., Coudiere, Y., Crystal, E., Ayache, N., Wright, Graham, A.: *In vivo* contact EP data and *ex vivo* MR-based computer models: registration and model-dependent errors. In: Camara, O., Mansi, T., Pop, M., Rhode, K., Sermesant, M., Young, A. (eds.) STACOM 2012. LNCS, vol. 7746, pp. 364–374. Springer, Heidelberg (2013). doi:10.1007/978-3-642-36961-2_41

10. Sermesant, M., Delingette, H., Ayache, N.: An electromechanical model of the heart for image analysis and simulations. IEEE Trans. Med. Imaging **25**(5), 612–625 (2006)

11. Aliev, R., Panfilov, A.V.: A simple two variables model of cardiac excitation. Chaos, Soliton Fractals **7**(3), 293–301 (1996)

12. Nash, M.P., Panfilov, A.V.: Electromechanical model of excitable tissue to study reentrant cardiac arrhythmias. Prog. Biophys. Mol. Biol. **85**, 501–522 (2004)

13. Keener, J.P., Sneeyd, J.: Mathematical Physiology. Spinger, New York (1998)

14. Talbot, H., Duriez, C., Courtecuisse, H., Relan, J., Sermesant, M., Cotin, S., Delingette, H.: Towards real-time computation of cardiac electrophysiology for training simulator. In: Camara, O., Mansi, T., Pop, M., Rhode, K., Sermesant, M., Young, A. (eds.) STACOM 2012. LNCS, vol. 7746, pp. 298–306. Springer, Heidelberg (2013). doi:10.1007/978-3-642-36961-2_34

15. Chinchapatnam, P., Rhode, K.S., Ginks, M., et al.: Model-based imaging of cardiac apparent conductivity and local conduction velocity for planning of therapy. IEEE Trans. Med. Imaging **27**(11), 1631–1642 (2008)

16. Li, Z., Athavale, P., Pop, M., Wright, G.A.: Multi-contrast reconstruction using compressed sensing with low rank and spatially-varying edge-preserving constraints for high-resolution MR characterization of myocardial infarction. Magn. Reson. Med. (September 2016, in press (Pubmed)). doi:10.1002/mrm.26402

Left Atrial Appendage Segmentation Based on Ranking 2-D Segmentation Proposals

Lei Wang, Jianjiang Feng$^{(\boxtimes)}$, Cheng Jin, Jiwen Lu, and Jie Zhou

Tsinghua National Laboratory for Information Science
and Technology Department of Automation, Tsinghua University, Beijing, China
{w-l14,jin-c12}@mails.tsinghua.edu.cn,
{jfeng,lujiwen,jzhou}@tsinghua.edu.cn

Abstract. The left atrial appendage (LAA) is the main source of thrombus in patients with atrial fibrillation (AF). Automated segmentation of the LAA can greatly help doctors diagnose thrombosis and plan LAA closure surgery. Considering large anatomical variations of the LAA, we present a non-model based semi-automated approach for LAA segmentation on CTA data. The method requires only manual selection of four fiducial points to obtain the bounding box for the LAA. Subsequently we generate a pool of segmentation proposals using parametric max-flow for each 2-D slice. Then a random forest regressor is trained to pick out the best 2-D proposal for each slice. Finally all selected 2-D proposals are merged into a 3-D model using spatial continuity. Experimental results on 60 CTA data showed that our approach was robust when dealing with large anatomical variations. Compared to manual annotation, we obtained an average dice overlap of 95.12%.

Keywords: Left atrial appendage · LAA closure surgery · Non-model based segmentation · Ranking

1 Introduction

Thrombosis has become a major contributor to the global disease burden [1]. International Society on Thrombosis and Haemostasis (ISTH) reported that one in four people worldwide die of conditions caused by thrombosis. The left atrial appendage (LAA) is the main source of thrombus in patients with atrial fibrillation (AF) [2]. The LAA is appended to the left atrium (LA) usually with an oval ostium (see Fig. 1(a)). It has several different complex morphologies named "windsock", "chicken wing", "cauliflower" and "cactus-like" with volume varying from 1 ml to 19 ml.

LAA morphology is related to the risk of thrombus in patients. The shape and size of the LAA may even change after AF and thrombosis. Doctors have to study the medical images carefully to diagnose pathological changes and thrombus in the LAA. Recently LAA closure surgery [3] has become a very promising treatment to prevent thrombosis. Due to complex LAA structure, doctors must know

© Springer International Publishing AG 2017
T. Mansi et al. (Eds.): STACOM 2016, LNCS 10124, pp. 21–29, 2017.
DOI: 10.1007/978-3-319-52718-5_3

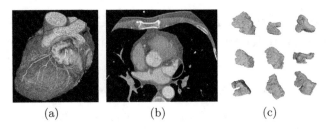

(a)   (b)   (c)

Fig. 1. The LAA. (a) Volume rendering of a heart with the LAA marked by green circle. (b) An axial CT slice with the LAA marked by green circle. (c) 3-D reconstruction models of 9 different LAAs from our data set. Shapes of LAAs vary significantly. (Color figure online)

LAA morphology and size exactly to plan surgery. Computed Tomography (CT) is widely used to visualize the heart anatomy before surgery. Automated LAA segmentation on CT data can greatly help doctors know the precise anatomical structure of the LAA in advance, which is very important for thrombosis treatment.

LAA segmentation on CT data is a quite challenging task due to the small size and large anatomical variations of the LAA. There is not too much work on LAA segmentation. Grasland-Mongrain et al. [4,5] used shape-constrained and inflation deformable models to segment the LAA, based on their previous heart segmentation framework [6]. They started from the segmented LA model, then grew the LAA model out using mesh inflation with shape constraints. It has some difficulties in segmenting the tip of the LAA [4,5] because of the constraints caused by the shape model. Zheng et al. [7] used a multi-part model to segment the whole LA, including the LAA in C-arm CT. The LAA has many small lobes but their boundaries are usually blurred in C-arm CT. Zheng et al. just used a smooth mesh to enclose all lobes roughly. Considering lobes are essential for modeling LAA morphology and they are clear in our Computed Tomography Angiography (CTA) data, unlike [7], we would include lobes into our segmentation work.

Model-based approaches [6,7] have been commonly used in medical image analysis. A series of work has obtained satisfactory results in heart chambers segmentation. Compared to heart chambers, the LAA has no significant shape prior due to large anatomical variations (see Fig. 1(c)). Thus non-model based approaches are preferred because they are purely driven by the image to be segmented without shape constraints. Graph-cut [8] is a widely used non-model based approach. However the value of parameter λ in Graph-cut has a strong impact on final result while it is a challenging task to determine the λ value. Instead of finding the optimal λ value, some work in computer vision [9,10] generated a pool of proposals using parametric max-flow/min-cut solver [11]. Parametric max-flow can solve max-flow/min-cut problem with a set of λ values while max-flow in Graph-cut just solves the problem with a single λ value.

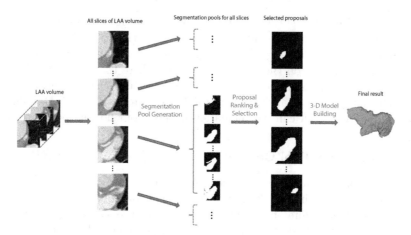

Fig. 2. Flowchart of our LAA segmentation algorithm. After LAA volume (a bounding box containing the LAA) is obtained by user interaction, we generate a pool of segmentation proposals for each axial slice. Then all proposals in each pool are ranked and the best one is selected for each slice. Finally we merge all selected 2-D proposals by spatial continuity to get the 3-D model.

After ranking the proposals in the pool, they achieved good performance in vision task like object segmentation.

In this paper, we proposed a three-step semi-automated approach to segment the LAA on CTA data. Figure 2 shows the framework of our approach. Considering large anatomical variations of the LAA, instead of using an explicit shape model, we rely on some general shape constraints, such as Gestalt features. Our approach achieved good performance with 95.12% average dice overlap when dealing with large anatomical variations of the LAA. Another major contribution of this paper is that in order to model LAA morphology exactly, we also segment LAA lobes precisely, which were not considered in [7].

2 Method

Considering large anatomical variations of the LAA and the difficulty of finding the optimal λ value in Graph-cut, we propose a non-model based semi-automated approach for LAA segmentation. The method only requires user to select four fiducial points to obtain a bounding box containing the LAA. Subsequently we use a three-step process (see Fig. 2) to segment the LAA:

- We generate a pool of segmentation proposals by setting different λ values and seed hypotheses for each axial slice.
- We rank the proposals in each pool based on some mid-level features and pick out the best proposal for each slice.
- We build the 3-D LAA model by merging the selected 2-D proposals and use spatial continuity of adjacent slices to correct possible segmentation errors.

User Interaction: As the LAA is just a small part of the whole CT volume, we require the user to mark a bounding box containing the LAA. The user should select four fiducial points around the LAA. One on the first axial slice where the LAA appears. Two on the middle axial slice where the area of the LAA is the largest, at the diagonal corners of a rectangle which can contain the LAA closely. One on the last axial slice where the LAA disappears. The 3-D bounding box containing the LAA can be calculated by these four fiducial points.

2.1   Segmentation Pool Generation

In this step, for each axial slice of the LAA (the reason why we choose axial slice will be explained in Sect. 3.1), we set different foreground and background seed hypotheses and different λ values to generate the segmentation pool. A segmentation pool is a series of proposals with high probability of including the good segmentations. For foreground seeds, we use sets of pixels that form small solid squares. Simpler than [10,12], we just place them automatically in rectangular grid geometry. For background seeds, we first use the set of pixels that cover full image borders. Whereas in a few slices the LAA is connected to the LA which covers the left and bottom borders, we also use the set of pixels that just cover the right and top borders. Figure 3 shows our seed hypotheses. For each seed hypothesis, we set 20 different λ values, ranging from 0 to 300.

Parametric max-flow can solve the above problem in the same complexity as the max-flow/min-cut problem with a single λ. It minimizes the energy with a set of λ values:

$$E^\lambda(\mathbf{x}) = \sum_{u \in \nu} U_\lambda(x_u) + \sum_{(u,v) \in \varepsilon} B_{uv}(x_u, x_v) . \tag{1}$$

The energy is a sum of unary term $U_\lambda(x_u)$ and binary term $B_{uv}(x_u, x_v)$. $\mathbf{x} = \{x_1, ..., x_u, ..., x_{|\nu|}\}$ is the label set defining a segmentation on the image while $x_u \in \{0, 1\}$ is the label assigned to the corresponding pixel u and $|\nu|$ equals to the number of pixels. 0 represents the background and 1 represents the foreground respectively. $G = (\nu, \varepsilon)$ is a graph with node set ν corresponding to image pixels and edge set ε encoding the similarity between neighboring pixels.

With a set of $\lambda \in \mathbb{R}$, the unary term is given as follows:

$$U_\lambda(x_u) = \begin{cases} 0 & \text{if } x_u = 1, u \notin \nu_b \\ \infty & \text{if } x_u = 1, u \in \nu_b \\ \infty & \text{if } x_u = 0, u \in \nu_f \\ f(x_u) + \lambda & \text{if } x_u = 0, u \notin \nu_f \end{cases} . \tag{2}$$

ν_b is the background-seed set while ν_f is the foreground-seed set. $f(x_u) + \lambda$ is the foreground bias and it represents the cost caused by assigning label 0 to the non foreground-seed pixels. $f(x_u) = lnp_f(u) - lnp_b(u)$ where $p_f(u) = \sum_k \pi_k \cdot N(I_u|\mu_k, \sigma_k)$ is the probability that pixel u belongs to foreground. Note that I_u is the grayscale of pixel u. $p_b(u)$ has the similar form.

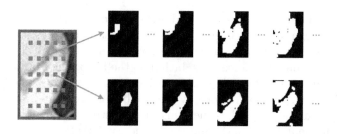

Fig. 3. Seed hypotheses. The small magenta squares represent different foreground seeds placed in rectangular grid. The bold blue lines at image borders represent background seeds. We also present the segmentation proposals for two different foreground seed hypotheses. In each set of proposals, λ increases from left to right. (Color figure online)

Binary term $B_{uv}(x_u, x_v)$ is the cost of assigning different labels to neighboring pixels:

$$B_{uv}(x_u, x_v) = \begin{cases} 0 & \text{if } x_u = x_v \\ A * exp(-\frac{(I_u - I_v)^2}{2\sigma^2}) \cdot \frac{1}{dist(u,v)} & \text{if } x_u \neq x_v \end{cases}. \qquad (3)$$

A is a scale factor and σ can be estimated as "camera noise" [8]. $dist(u, v)$ is the distance of pixel u and pixel v.

And in this paper, the algorithm in [11] is used as the parametric max-flow solver.

2.2 Proposal Ranking and Selection

We aim to pick out the proposals having high ground truth overlap in each pool. One feasible method is introducing a ranker to rank all proposals and keeping the top one as the finally picked proposal. We cast the problem of ranking proposals as regression on quality measure of proposals against their segmented image features. Random forest is used as our regressor. And we use the **Dice overlap** as the quality measure. The Dice overlap between two regions R and R' is defined:

$$\mathcal{D}(R, R') = \frac{2|R \cap R'|}{|R| + |R'|}. \qquad (4)$$

Two kinds of features are used to describe each proposal: the region features and the Gestalt features. Region features encode the statistics of the position, scale and shape of the segmented region. They consist of 17 features in total, including the relative position to the image center, the relative area to the image area, the lengths of the major and minor axis of the ellipse that has the same normalized second central moments as the region, the relative distance between the extrema points in the region and the image center to the image size, ratio of pixels in the region to pixels in the bounding box tightly containing the region, proportion of the pixels in the convex hull that are also in the region, and

Euler number. Gestalt features are mid-level cues encoding the convexity and continuity properties. Psychologists argue that Gestalt features like convexity, continuity and symmetry are important for visual grouping [13]. In our paper, Gestalt features consist of 6 features, including the histogram of the foreground region, relative intra-region edge energy which is the sum of the edge energy inside the foreground region divided by the number of foreground pixels, relative inter-region edge energy which is the sum of the edge energy along the boundary divided by the boundary length, and the boundary curvature.

2.3   3-D Model Building Using Spatial Continuity

After picking out the best proposal for each slice, all the selected 2-D proposals can be directly merged into a 3-D model. However, the continuity and consistency between adjacent slices are ignored while they are useful to improve the quality of the 3-D model. In object tracking, time continuity which is the strong correlation between adjacent frames is a very important cue. While in our task, the segmentation results of the adjacent slices are related to each other, which we call spatial continuity. We take 3 adjacent slices into account. For the current slice, we check the segmentation results of its former and latter slices to recover the missing disconnected components of the LAA and correct the small leakage to neighboring anatomical structures. Besides spatial continuity, we also use mathematical morphology including eroding and dilating to improve the quality of the final result.

3   Experiments

3.1   Data Set and Manual Annotation

We randomly selected our data set from patients who underwent a CTA examination using a Philips Brilliance iCT256 scanner from August 2015 to December 2015. The volumes in our data set may contain 235 to 713 slices while the size of all slices is of 512×512 pixels. The resolution inside each slice is isotropic but varies between 0.314 mm and 0.508 mm for different volumes. The slice thickness is the same with 0.450 mm for all volumes.

Phase and Slice Selection. The original data set has four phases for each patient with 40% and 45% in electrical systole and 70% and 78% in electrical diastole. Since the image quality is similar among these phases, we chose 45% phase because according to [2] the LAA at this phase has a big volume. We prefer 2-D slices to 3-D volume mainly because we can parallel the segmentation pool generation step which is the most time-consuming with 2-D slices processed independently. Axial slices are chosen because sagittal and coronal slices are no better for studying LAA morphology [3] while the number of slices in axial plane is much fewer.

Ground Truth Annotation. With the help of radiologists, we annotated the LAA using a paint brush tool [14] slice by slice at the voxel level. The annotations were mainly done at axial slices and corrected by checking sagittal and coronal slices. In a few slices where the LAA is connected to the LA, a small part of the LA inside the region of interest was also included in the LAA.

3.2 Results

We evaluated our approach on 60 CTA data and used a four-fold cross-validation to measure the LAA segmentation quality. The random forest was trained on 45 CTA data and tested on the last 15. Table 1 shows the results of our experiment. To evaluate step 1, we measured the quality of the segmentation pool with average best dice overlap presented. Average best dice overlap is the mean dice value of the best proposals in all pools. To evaluate step 2 (proposal ranking), we reported the dice value of top 1 proposal, the mean dice values of top 5 proposals and bottom 5 proposals. The quality of top 5 and bottom 5 proposals demonstrated that the results of our ranker were quite reasonable. After the final step, we obtained an average dice overlap of 95.12%. The method took about 3.5 min for a LAA volume, with about 3 min for the segmentation pool generation step, on 4 Intel Core i7 processors at 4.0 GHz with 16 GB of RAM.

Previous work [4,5] used a model-based approach to segment the LAA. Testing the approach on 17 CT data, they obtained an average dice overlap of 70.81%, max dice overlap of 85.42% and min dice overlap of 16.58% while ours are 95.12%, 98.83%, and 81.16%. As mentioned in [4,5], their model-based approach has difficulties in segmenting LAA tip and lobes because of large anatomical variations. The results showed that our non-model based approach did not suffer from this problem. We did not compare our results with [7] because the lobes were not considered in [7].

Table 1. The dice overlap after each step of our approach

	Pool quality	Ranked proposals			Final result
		Top 1	Top 5	Bottom 5	
Dice	0.9467	0.9120	0.8954	0.100	0.9512

Figure 4 presents the results of two examples. It shows that our approach can generate segmentation pools with high quality (see column 1 of each example) and our ranker can pick out the best proposal in most cases (see column 2 of each example). Although in a few cases the ranker failed to pick the correct proposal out, step 3 successfully recovered the missing components (see row 2 of example 1) and corrected the leakage to neighboring anatomical structures (see row 3 of example 2).

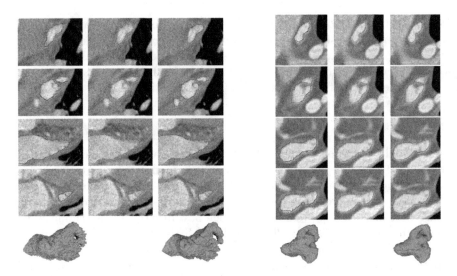

Fig. 4. Segmentation results of two examples. Left: example 1. Right: example 2. For each example, column 1–3: the results after step 1–3 of our approach, row 1–4: 4 different axial slices and row 5: the model reconstructed from the ground truth (left) and the model reconstructed by our approach (right). Red curves represent the ground truth while blue, cyan and green curves show the best proposals in segmentation pools, picked proposals and the final results respectively. Step 1 can generate pools with high quality and step 2 is able to pick out good proposals generally. Step 3 can recover the missing components (see row 2 of example 1), correct the leakage to neighboring structures (see row 3 of example 2), and make the final shapes smoother (see row 5 of example 1). (Color figure online)

4   Conclusion

In this paper, we propose a non-model based semi-automated approach for segmenting the LAA, including the LAA tip and lobes. The approach is based on learning to rank 2-D segmentation proposals. The experiment showed that our approach was robust in dealing with large anatomical variations. We obtained an average dice overlap of 95.12% on 60 CTA data, much better than previously reported LAA segmentation accuracy (70.81%) [5].

A limitation of current approach is that it requires manual selection of four fiducial points to obtain the bounding box for the LAA. One way to address this problem is to segment the LA chamber first. As the LAA is appended to the LA chamber, it should be convenient to locate the LAA automatically by extending the segmented LA chamber.

Acknowledgements. This work is supported by the National Natural Science Foundation of China under Grants 61225008, 61373074, 61572271, 61527808 and 61373090, the National Basic Research Program of China under Grant 2014CB349304, the Ministry of Education of China under Grant 20120002110033, and the Tsinghua University Initiative Scientific Research Program.

References

1. Rosendaal, F.R., Raskob, G.E.: On world thrombosis day. The Lancet **384**(9955), 1653–1654 (2014)
2. Patti, G., Pengo, V., et al. The left atrial appendage: from embryology to prevention of thromboembolism. Eur. Heart J. doi: http://dx.doi.org/10.1093/eurheartj/ehw159. Epub 2016 Apr 26
3. Wang, Y., Di Biase, L., et al.: Left atrial appendage studied by computed tomography to help planning for appendage closure device placement. J. Cardiovasc. Electrophysiol. **21**(9), 973–982 (2010)
4. Grasland-Mongrain, P., Peters, J., Ecabert, O.: Combination of shape-constrained and inflation deformable models with application to the segmentation of the left atrial appendage. In: ISBI, pp. 428–431 (2010)
5. Grasland-Mongrain, P.: Segmentation of the left atrial appendage from 3D images. Master Thesis. ENS Cachan (2009)
6. Ecabert, O., Peters, J., Schramm, H., Lorenz, C., et al.: Automatic model-based segmentation of the heart in CT images. IEEE Trans. Med. Imaging **27**(9), 1189–1201 (2008)
7. Zheng, Y., Yang, D., John, M., Comaniciu, D.: Multi-part modeling and segmentation of left atrium in C-arm CT for image-guided ablation of atrial fibrillation. IEEE Trans. Med. Imaging **33**(2), 318–331 (2014)
8. Boykov, Y., Funka-Lea, G.: Graph cuts and efficient N-D image segmentation. Int. J. Comput. Vis. **70**(2), 109–131 (2006)
9. Kolmogorov, V., Boykov, Y., Rother, C.: Applications of parametric maxflow in computer vision. In: ICCV 2007, pp. 1–8 (2007)
10. Carreira, J., Sminchisescu, C.: CPMC: automatic object segmentation using constrained parametric min-cuts. IEEE Trans. Pattern Anal. Mach. Intell. **34**(7), 1312–1328 (2012)
11. Hochbaum, D.S.: The pseudoflow algorithm: a new algorithm for the maximum-flow problem. Oper. Res. **56**(4), 992–1009 (2008)
12. Carreira, J., Sminchisescu, C.: Constrained parametric min-cuts for automatic object segmentation, release 1. http://sminchisescu.ins.uni-bonn.de/code/cpmc/
13. Wertheimer, M.: Laws of organization in perceptual forms (partial translation). In: A Source-Book of Gestalt Psycychology, pp. 71–88 (1938)
14. Fedorov, A., Beichel, R., et al.: 3D slicer as an image computing platform for the quantitative imaging network. Magn. Reson. Imaging **30**(9), 1323–1341 (2012)

Correction of Slice Misalignment
in Multi-breath-hold Cardiac MRI Scans

Benjamin Villard[1(✉)], Ernesto Zacur[1], Erica Dall'Armellina[2],
and Vicente Grau[1]

[1] Institute of Biomedical Engineering, University of Oxford, Oxford, UK
`benjamin.villard@eng.ox.ac.uk`
[2] Division of Cardiovascular Medicine, Radcliffe Department of Medicine,
Oxford Acute Vascular Imaging Center, University of Oxford, Oxford, UK

Abstract. Cardiac Magnetic Resonance (CMR) provides unique functional and anatomical visualisation of the macro and micro-structures of the heart. However, CMR acquisition times usually necessitate slices to be acquired at different breath holds, which results in potential misalignment of the acquired slices. Correcting for this spatial misalignment is required for accurate three-dimensional (3D) reconstruction of the heart chambers allowing robust metrics for shape analysis among populations as well as precise representations of individual geometries and scars. While several methods have been proposed to realign slices, their use in other important protocols such as late gadolinium enhancement (LGE) is yet to be demonstrated. We propose a registration framework based on local phase to correct for slice misalignment. Our registration framework is a group registration technique combining long- and short-axis slices. Validation was performed on LGE slices using expert-traced ventricular contours. For 15 clinical multi-breath-hold datasets our method reduced the median discrepancy of moderately misaligned slices from 2.19 mm to 1.63 mm, and of severely misaligned from 7.33 mm to 1.96 mm.

Keywords: Slice misalignment · Late gadolinium enhancement · CMR

1 Introduction

Cardiovascular diseases are one of the world's biggest killers, accounting for over 4 million deaths in Europe yearly [1]. Enabling early diagnosis and effective treatment is essential to the reduction of the burden of cardiovascular diseases.

In recent years much research has looked at creating personalised 3D anatomical models of the heart [2]. These models usually incorporate a geometrical reconstruction of the anatomy in order to understand better cardiovascular functions as well as predict different processes after a clinical event. Also, population studies of cardiac anatomy require precise geometrical reconstructions [3,4]. However the ability to accurately reconstruct heart anatomy from MRI in three dimensions commonly comes with a fundamental challenge: the misalignment

© Springer International Publishing AG 2017
T. Mansi et al. (Eds.): STACOM 2016, LNCS 10124, pp. 30–38, 2017.
DOI: 10.1007/978-3-319-52718-5_4

between slices acquired at different breath holds. In this paper we discuss an alignment algorithm for individual CMR slices that allows subsequent accurate reconstruction of geometrical models of the heart. The algorithm uses the intersection lines between slices, introducing a new cost function designed to be applied on both cine and late gadolinium images, as well as a specifically designed optimisation strategy. The main contributions of this work are:

- The development of a complete framework for the correction of translational and rotational misalignments between CMR slices, based on the combination of short axes (SA) and long axes (LA) images and applicable to cine and LGE CMR scans.
- The introduction of the normalised cross correlation of local phase vectors as a similarity measure that makes the method applicable to different CMR protocols.
- A complete validation using manually traced contours, which includes the estimation of contouring errors.

1.1   Misalignment Between CMR Slices

CMR images allow for detailed ventricular anatomical information as well as an accurate representation of myocardial function by using a plethora of available specialised protocols. Acquiring cardiac images is a complex process due to the constant motion of the heart. Standard clinical protocols do not allow 3D images of the heart in a single acquisition, and thus typically acquire a collection of 2D slices, oriented either on the short axis or on a long axis plane of the ventricles, each one at a separate breath hold. Electrocardiogram (ECG) allow the images to compensate for cardiac motion. Breath holding at the same lung volume for periods ranging from 7 to 15 s is used to reduce slice misalignment from the acquisition. This alignment distortion may be further enhanced by any patient movement inside the scanner, affecting slice spatial coherence as a 3D dataset [5].

1.2   Motion Correction

A significant amount of research has been dedicated to the correction of CMR slice misalignment. Some studies solely align endo and epicardial contours with regards to each other. This requires the availability of accurate contours, and has the disadvantage of forfeiting all the additional information available in the image values. In practice, due to the inter/intra variability in expert contouring, the final alignment will depend on the expert; on the other hand, if the application requires the smoothest ventricular shapes possible, methods such as [6] can be used. Other studies use volumetric approaches where individual slices are registered to a 3D volume (slice-to-volume registration) [7–9]. The second common approach in the literature uses slice-to-slice alignment (slice-to slice registration), which is also used in our method. This approach is based on using the image intensities at the slice intersections. By optimising over the (dis)similarity between intensities on the intersecting line, optimal alignment can be achieved.

Some studies [10,11] use a fixed slice, usually an LA slice, to which all the other slices are aligned to. The drawback to this is the dependence on the choice of the reference slice, which can heavily influence the results if a particularly misaligned slice is chosen as the fixed reference. An alternative method is to alternate the reference slice in an iterative manner and allow the other slices to register to it. This has the negative effect of being highly influenced by outliers and makes the process more sensitive to local minima. This results in optimising over a space of $6n$ parameters, with n being the number of slices, which is costly and less efficient. To minimize the amount of local minima, our method fixes all the other slices and allows only one slice to "move", obtaining the best *global* alignment. Furthermore using the sum of similarity measures from a slice to several reference slices can lower the influence of outliers, forcing them to converge through an iterative process; also known as alternate optimisation [12]. Theoretically, different alignment strategies could converge to the same minimum, regardless of the optimisation parameters used. However, the presence of local minima means that, in practice, the choice of optimisation parameters has a substantial effect on the result.

1.3   Similarity Function

Cost functions, otherwise known as similarity measures, provide a measure of (dis)similarity between images/intensities in the domain of image registration. Similarity functions can be feature-based, which aim at the alignment of specific image features (e.g. edges), or voxel-based, which use all intensity values and quantifies their differences. Voxel-based measures can usually be posed in a generative and statistical framework providing a measure of mutual dependence between random variables. The similarity criterion is one of the key factors in the performance of a registration process, and depends on the nature of the data to be registered [13]. Protocols including gadolinium injections suffer from contrast wash-in/wash-out in the images, increasing the disparity in intensities between slices at different time instants. This prevents the use of simple measures based on intensity differences, such as Sum of Absolute/Square Differences (SAD/SSD). Although some studies such as [14] use SSD as a similarity function, they only apply to same plane (2D-2D) registration, whereas in our case, the intensity discrepancy mostly occurs between the LA and SA slices. We consider that the use of a contrast-independent measure based on salient features would be more appropriate to match the line intersection profiles. Phase based metrics have been a popular choice to use in the last years [15,16]. Local phase is a contrast independent descriptor of image structure and is thus not affected by intensity discrepancies [17].

2   Materials and Methods

2.1   CMR Data

The datasets used consists of DICOM files containing 2D CINE MRI and 2D LGE sequences of size 216×256 pixels (approx: $1.41\,\text{mm} \times 1.41\,\text{mm}$). 15 datasets

(SIEMENS TrioTim 3 T scanner at the John Radcliffe Hospital, Oxford, UK) from different subjects were used. Each dataset contains between 9 and 13 SA slices from apex to base separated by 8/10 mm and 3 LA slices (4 chamber view, 2 chamber view and out-flow tract). For validation purposes, left ventricle epi- and endocardial contours were manually traced by an expert on all SA and LA slices using the CMR42 software (Circle Cardiovascular Imaging, Calgary, Canada).

2.2 Image Registration Algorithm

Our method relies on the intensity profiles at the line formed by the intersection between two slices to align the slices together and give spatial coherence to the 3D dataset. This is based on the assumption that two slices will be perfectly aligned when the underlying features of the line profile at their intersection is complementary. Assuming that slices from a subject are triggered at the same cardiac phase the 3D shape/anatomy of the heart remains fixed among slices. Therefore, rigid-body transformations between slices are considered. As such, we perform rigid registration for each of the slices over 6° of freedom of a rigid-body transformation (Fig. 1).

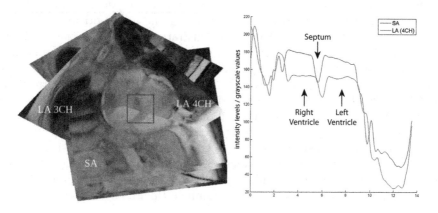

Fig. 1. Left panel shows some 2D MRI slices in their spatial 3D positions, where a clear misalignment can be shown (red box). Right panel shows the intensity profiles along an intersection line. (Color figure online)

2.3 Alignment Score and Optimisation Strategy

The global motion (GM) discrepancy of the slices can be measured as the sum of (dis)similarity measures E between pair of intersecting slices. Let S_i be the i-th slice and Θ_i the set of its 6 rigid transformation parameters, for example $\Theta = \{t_x, t_y, t_z, \alpha, \beta, \gamma\}$ (in our case 3 translations plus 3 Euler angles). Moreover, let $S_i^{\Theta_i}$ be the transformed version of the slice S_i by the rigid transformation defined by parameters Θ_i. By using this notation, the global motion (GM) discrepancy is given by

$$GM\left(\Theta_1, \Theta_2, \ldots, \Theta_n; S_1, S_2, \ldots, S_n\right) = \sum E\left(S_i^{\Theta_i}, S_j^{\Theta_j}\right) \tag{1}$$

where the summation runs over all pairs S_i, S_j intersecting in a line, *i.e.* an LA slice will intersect with all the SAs and the other LAs. Minimising GM is akin to finding the parameters for each slice. In this work, this minimisation is performed in an alternate manner, by optimising the parameters Θ of a single slice whilst leaving the others fixed. As the GM is built as a sum of terms, the iterative minimisation of partial terms results in the minimisation of the global motion discrepancy and the slices match together.

2.4   Similarity Measure

The particularities of image acquisition described in Sect. 2.1 prevent the use of simple measures based on intensity differences, such as SAD/SSD. For images with high intensity disparity, feature-based similarity measure can provide a more robust method of assessing similarity between the images at the intersection profiles. As local phase is independent of contrast and not affected by intensity inconsistencies, it is a sensible choice as a similarity measure. The local phase can be obtained through the analytic signal in 1D, and general extensions to higher dimensions have been proposed including the use of oriented filters or the monogenic signal [16]. Although our registration is based on the similarity between the 1D intersecting line profiles, we compute the local phase for an entire image, and then obtain the line intersection between two local phase images as it results in less noise in the line profiles [16]. The normalised cross correlation (NCC) between two profiles is used as similarity measure E for an intersecting pair. In 2D, the local frequency information can be obtained by convolving the images with banks of quadrature pairs of log-Gabor filters [15]. A quadrature filter is a complex valued function which transforms a real valued signal to an analytical signal with weighted frequency components. Convolving the image with a filter will result in response vectors encoding phase and amplitude. By using quadrature filters, local phase (Φ) can be estimated by

$$\Phi = \arctan\left(\frac{I_q}{I_p}\right) \tag{2}$$

where I_q represents the magnitude of the odd filters convolved with the image, and I_p the filter response. With respect to 2D, quadrature filters can be generalised through directional formulation [18]. This results in the image that can be seen in Fig. 3. Once the local phase images are obtained, the line intersection at both images is taken to account for the similarity measure, using NCC.

2.5   Contour-Based Alignment

Due to inconsistencies in manual contouring of the SA and LA slices, a "perfect" alignment (i.e. one in which the distances between SA and LA contour is zero) might not be achievable. In order to establish a baseline error value, we applied a misalignment correction algorithm using the contours from manual images, substituting function E() in Eq. (1) by the Euclidean distance between SA and LA contours. We refer to this algorithm as "contour-based" to differentiate it from the "image-based" algorithm we propose here.

3   Results

We investigated the performance of the registration algorithm using the normalised correlation of the local phase signals. The algorithm was used on 15 datasets, each containing 3 LAs and several SAs. The algorithm was run for 9 iterations, for each dataset, in order to evaluate the convergence of the registration. This number was chosen empirically, as the algorithm appeared to converge by then (see Fig. 2).

Table 1 shows the mean, median, and standard deviation resulting from contour to contour distance calculations before the alignment and after, using the image based method, and contour only method. The upper part of the table represents all of the 682 individual contour to contour distance for all the datasets. The lower part reports the values for the 82 contours that were deemed significantly misaligned (>5 mm).

Table 1. Top: LGE phase results for all 15 patients before alignment and after 9 different iterations, as well as with alignment by minimising contours only. Bottom: Same as above but for significantly misaligned slices.

	Before	Image based	Contour based
Median:	2.19	1.63	0.31
Mean:	2.82	2.03	0.46
Std:	2.48	1.71	0.47
Median:	7.33	1.96	0.29
Mean:	7.73	2.72	0.43
Std:	2.43	2.36	0.44

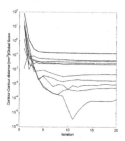

Fig. 2. Pairwise energy E between slices over several iterations. Red line shows the global energy GM. (Color figure online)

4   Discussion

Our method relies on using all available information to correct for misalignment by using both the long and short axes slices, in an iterative process. By taking into account all intersections simultaneously, we minimize the effect that individual outliers have on the overall results, forcing these outliers towards the global "consensus" position. By using local phase, we rely on its invariance to changes

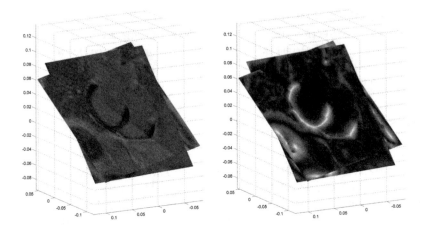

Fig. 3. Late gadolinium image on the left and local phase image on the right

of intensities in order to focus on obtaining high feature similarity rather than high intensity profile similarity. Relying on the latter assumes that the images to be registered contain similar intensity profiles which is not always the case.

The slice optimisation was constrained to compensate for potential structural symmetry, which might lead to out of plane misalignment such as could be the case with midventricle short axis slices. A hard constraint was chosen as an alternative to introducing a regulariser as the latter would induce a bias towards the initial positions of the planes.

The median and mean values for all 15 patients can be observed to decrease notably, however our method distinguishes itself more with regards to the remarkably misaligned slices. We have defined significantly misaligned slices as slices having higher than 5 mm between contours. Results show that the median value before the alignment is 7.33 mm (7.73 mm mean). After the alignment, a median of 1.96 mm was obtained (2.72 mm mean). By minimising the contour to contour distances only, results show that zero minimal distance is unobtainable, due to the variability in contouring. As such, the lowest median obtainable with our contours was 0.29 mm (0.43 mm mean), which should be accounted for when looking at the image based results.

Oscillations along the iterations of the alternate optimisation are a concern due to the slice dependencies. This can be observed in the behaviour of the global energy at the different iterations (see Fig. 2). It can be seen empirically that 10–20 iterations are enough to converge. GM can be seen to decrease and follow a descent path without any jumps occurring, however the evolution of the pairwise energy can result in a non-monotonic (non-descent) path. Even after running the algorithm for more then 100 iterations, some energy pairs will continue oscillating. It can also be seen that for a given pair, the lower the energy, the more it oscillates.

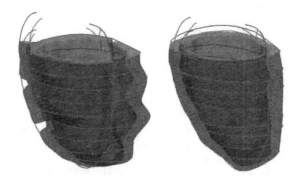

Fig. 4. Surface reconstruction before and after alignment.

Validation for cardiac image processing comes with some important drawbacks that need to be taken into account. There typically exist no true ground truth due to the nature of the problems. In the majority of cases the ground truth relies on quantification values based on clinical segmentation. However expert segmentation should not be considered as the true ground truth, but more as an approximation, as it suffers from inter-intra expert variability. Furthermore the choice of quantification methods is highly variable and can greatly impact the results.

It can be said that the motion correction algorithm is indispensable for any cardiac anatomical reconstruction which is clearly shown by Fig. 4. Several artifacts can be observed such as non aligned SA contours causing a "waving" surface. Furthermore spatial discrepancies between SAs and LAs produces depth fissures and ridges of the surfaces and discrepancies between LAs do not allow for a good reconstruction of the apical region.

We have presented a phase based registration algorithm that corrects for the misalignment of LGE MRI images. This framework will be used as a preprocessing step in 3D reconstructions of the heart, leading to accurate anatomical models.

Acknowledgments. BV acknowledges the support of the RCUK Digital Economy Programme grant number EP/G036861/1 (Oxford Centre for Doctoral Training in Healthcare Innovation). EZ acknowledges the Marie Sklodowska-Curie Individual Fellowship from the H2020 EU Framework Programme for Research and Innovation [Proposal No: 655020-DTI4micro-MSCA-IF-EF-ST]. ED acknowledges the BHF intermediate clinical research fellow grant (FS/13/71/30378) and the NIHR BRC. VG is supported by a BBSRC grant (BB/I012117/1), an EPSRC grant (EP/J013250/1) and by BHF New Horizon Grant NH/13/30238.

References

1. escardio.org. European Cardiovascular Disease Statistics 2012 (2012)
2. Arevalo, H.J., Vadakkumpadan, F., Guallar, E., Jebb, A., Malamas, P., Wu, K.C., Trayanova, N.A.: Arrhythmia risk stratification of patients after myocardial infarction using personalized heart models. Nat. Commun. **7** (2016)
3. Lamata, P., Sinclair, M., Kerfoot, E., Lee, A., Crozier, A., Blazevic, B., Land, S., Lewandowski, A.J., Barber, D., Niederer, S.: An automatic service for the personalization of ventricular cardiac meshes. J. R. Soc. Interface **11**(91) (2013)
4. Young, A.A., Frangi, A.F.: Computational cardiac atlases: from patient to population and back. Exp. Physiol. **94**(5), 578–596 (2009)
5. Bogaert, J., Dymarkowski, S., Taylor, A.M., Muthurangu, V.: Clinical Cardiac MRI. Springer, Heidelberg (2012)
6. Su, Y., Tan, M.-L., Lim, C.-W., Teo, S.-K., Tan, R.-S., Wan, M., Selvaraj, S.K.: Automatic correction of motion artifacts in 4D left ventricle model reconstructed from MRI. In: Computing in Cardiology 2014, vol. 41, pp. 705–708 (2014)
7. Chandler, A.G., Pinder, R.J., Netsch, T., Schnabel, J.A., Hawkes, D.J., Hill, D.L.G., Razavi, R.: Correction of misaligned slices in multi-slice cardiovascular magnetic resonance using slice-to-volume registration. J. Cardiovasc. Magn. Reson. **10**(1), 1–9 (2008)
8. Zakkaroff, C., Radjenovic, A., Greenwood, J., Magee, D.: Stack alignment transform for misalignment correction in cardiac MR cine series. Technical report, University of Leeds (2012)
9. Lotjonen, J., Pollari, M., Kivisto, S., Lauerma, K.: Correction of movement artifacts from 4-D cardiac short- and long-axis MR data. In: International Conference on Medical Image Computing and Computer-Assisted Intervention, pp. 405–412 (2004)
10. Goshtasby, A.A., Turner, D.A.: Fusion of short-axis and long-axis cardiac MR images. In: Proceedings of the Workshop on Mathematical Methods in Biomedical Image Analysis, 1996, pp. 202–211, June 1996
11. McLeish, K., Hill, D.L.G., Atkinson, D., Blackall, J.M., Razavi, R.: A study of the motion and deformation of the heart due to respiration. IEEE Trans. Med. Imaging **21**(9), 1142–1150 (2002)
12. Bezdek, J.C., Hathaway, R.J.: Convergence of alternating optimization. Neural, Parallel Sci. Comput. **11**(4), 351–368 (2003)
13. Perperidis, D.: Spatio-temporal registration and modelling of the heart using cardiovascular MR imaging. Ph.D. thesis, Imperial College London (2006)
14. Ledesma-Carbayo, M.J., Kellman, P., Arai, A.E., McVeigh, E.R.: Motion corrected free-breathing delayed-enhancement imaging of myocardial infarction using non-rigid registration. J. Magn. Reson. Imaging **26**(1), 184–190 (2007)
15. Kovesi, P.: Image features from phase congruency. Videre: J. Comput. Vis. Res. **1**(3), 1–26 (1999)
16. Bernstein, S., Bouchot, J.-L., Reinhardt, M., Heise, B.: Generalized analytic signals in image processing: comparison, theory and applications. In: Hitzer, E., Sangwine, S.J. (eds.) Quaternion and Clifford Fourier Transforms and Wavelets. Trends in Mathematics, pp. 221–246. Springer, Basel (2013)
17. Kelly, C., Neubauer, S., Choudhury, R., Dall'Armellina, E., Grau, V.: A local phase-based algorithm for registration of CMR scans from multiple visits. In: Computing in Cardiology 2014, pp. 937–940. IEEE (2014)
18. Derpanis, K.G.: Quadrature Filters. Department of Computer Science and Engineering, York University (2005)

Phase-Based Registration of Cardiac Tagged MR Images by Incorporating Anatomical Constraints

Yitian Zhou[1,3]([⊠]), Mathieu De Craene[1],
Maxime Sermesant[2], and Olivier Bernard[3]

[1] Philips Research Medisys, Suresnes, France
yitian.zhou@philips.com
[2] Inria, Asclepios Research Project, Sophia Antipolis, France
[3] CREATIS, CNRS UMR5220, Inserm U1044, INSA-Lyon,
Université Lyon 1, Villeurbanne, France

Abstract. This paper presents a novel method that combines respective benefits of the tracking-based methods and the Gabor-based non-tracking approaches for improving the motion/strain quantification from tagged MR images. The "tag number constant" concept used in Gabor-based non-tracking methods is integrated into a recent phase-based registration framework. We evaluated our method on both synthetic and real data: (1) on a synthetic data of a normal heart, we found that the constraint improved both longitudinal and circumferential strains accuracies; (2) on 15 healthy volunteers, the proposed method achieved better tracking accuracy compared to three state-of-the-art methods; (3) on one patient dataset, we show that our method is able to distinguish the infarcted segments from the normal ones.

Keywords: Cardiac tagged MR · Strain · Tag number constant constraint

1 Introduction

The quantification of regional myocardial motion and strains remains a central challenge for diagnosing heart diseases. Tagged magnetic resonance imaging (TMRI) is currently the gold standard for quantifying local myocardial deformations. The underlying technique is based on the creation of non-invasive magnetic markers (tags) that move with the myocardium over the cardiac cycle. Tracking these tags permits the recovery of underlying cardiac deformations.

As for the state-of-the-art on cardiac motion tracking from TMRI, the reader is referred to [1] for a thorough analysis. We provide here a brief discussion relevant to this paper. All the developed algorithms can be roughly classified into two categories: the tracking-based and the Gabor-based non-tracking methods. The tracking-based methods consist in (1) tracking the myocardial motion by HARP [2], optical flow or any other non-rigid registration technique and (2) deriving the strain from the tracked field. One limitation of such methods is that

© Springer International Publishing AG 2017
T. Mansi et al. (Eds.): STACOM 2016, LNCS 10124, pp. 39–47, 2017.
DOI: 10.1007/978-3-319-52718-5_5

the computed strain is highly sensitive to the regularization parameter used for the tracking [3]. As a result, Qian *et al.* [3], Bruurmijn *et al.* [4] and Kause *et al.* [5] opted for bypassing the tracking issue. They proposed to directly compute Eulerian strain maps from spatial tag frequencies that were filtered out by Gabor filters. The idea is that temporal variations in spatial tag frequencies reveals the stretch/shortening of the myocardium. For example, an increased spatial tag frequency means that the tissue undergoes a local contraction. All of the above groups made use of this concept to compute the deformation gradient tensor which is further related to strain. They all used the assumption that the **N**umber of **T**ags between two myocardial points remains **C**onstant over the cardiac cycle (denoted as NTC hereinafter). This assumption is implicit in [3] while explicit in both [4,5]. The authors claim that it makes their strain estimate independent to any tracking field. However, they overlook that a tracking is always required for reporting strain evolution at all time points per material point, which is of clinical importance in diagnosing heart diseases like dyssynchrony, infarction *etc.*

In this paper, we propose to integrate the NTC into a recent phase-based registration framework [6]. By exploiting NTC as constraints defined in the anatomical directions of the heart, we aim to reduce the dependency of the strain output to the amount of regularization and report strain curves per material point. The constraints are used as an additional step for refining the tracking of myocardial points located in the middle of the myocardium. The role the NTC plays in improving the quantification is evaluated on both synthetic and real data.

2   Data Acquisition and Preprocessing

A full description of the acquisition of the TMRI used can be found in [1]. The data consists of three sequences with orthogonal tagging directions. In the following, the sequence is identified by the index k ($k = 0, 1, 2$).

We follow the preprocessing steps described in [1]. It consists of (1) the computation of HARP phase; (2) the manual segmentation of the left ventricle (LV) at end-diastole and its resampling to a volumetric mesh. The resampled mesh has three layers in the radial direction: endocardium (endo), epicardium (epi) and a middle layer located between them (mid); and (3) the division of LV domain into local windows according to the AHA standard. The apex segment (n° 17) was further subdivided into three equal parts, resulting in 19 windows in total. Gaussian window functions (Fig. 2(b)) were then defined for each window.

3   Methodology

We chose to track each of the endo/mid/epi layers independently (This choice is justified later in Sect. 3.1). First, we track each of the endo/epi/mid layers by the purely phase-based registration (Sect. 3.2) using a recent parametric motion model (Sect. 3.1). Second, we refine the motion of the mid layer using the phase-based registration with NTC constraints (Sect. 3.3). We chose not to refine the endo and epi layers because they subject to tracking artifacts which impact the computation of accurate number of tags that we impose as constraints. The way we implement the NTC constraint is later detailed in Sect. 3.3.

3.1   Motion Model

We use the parametric model proposed in [1] to represent the motion. With the acquisition protocol used, there is a poor tag resolution in the radial direction (only 2 or 3 line tags), making it difficult to capture accurate transmural motion variations [1]. As a result, we decided to remove the three parameters that represent the transmural gradients of *Rad.*, *Long.* and *Circ.* (RLC) displacements from the model. This leads to a 9-parameter model per window per layer:

$$\mathbf{v}(\mathbf{x}) = \sum_i \varphi^{(i)}(\mathbf{x})\mathbf{v}^{(i)}(\mathbf{x})$$

$$\text{with } \mathbf{v}^{(i)}(\mathbf{x}) = \left(a_{rl}^{(i)}l^{(i)}(\mathbf{x}) + a_{rc}^{(i)}c^{(i)}(\mathbf{x}) + b_r^{(i)}\right)\hat{\mathbf{e}}_r(\mathbf{x}) + \\ \left(a_{ll}^{(i)}l^{(i)}(\mathbf{x}) + a_{lc}^{(i)}c^{(i)}(\mathbf{x}) + b_l^{(i)}\right)\hat{\mathbf{e}}_l(\mathbf{x}) + \\ \left(a_{cl}^{(i)}l^{(i)}(\mathbf{x}) + a_{cc}^{(i)}c^{(i)}(\mathbf{x}) + b_c^{(i)}\right)\rho(\mathbf{x})\hat{\mathbf{e}}_c(\mathbf{x}) \quad (1)$$

where $\mathbf{v}^{(i)}$ is the local motion inside the window i, $\varphi^{(i)}$ are Gaussian window functions, and $\mathbf{v}$ is the global motion that results from mixing local motions. $\hat{\mathbf{e}}_d(\mathbf{x})$ $(d = r, l, c)$ are RLC directions. $l^{(i)}$ and $c^{(i)}$ are local coordinates along *Long.* and *Circ.* directions respectively. ρ is the distance to the long axis [1]. In this way, $\{b_r^{(i)}, b_l^{(i)}, b_c^{(i)}\}$ represent translations, $\{a_{ll}^{(i)}, a_{cc}^{(i)}\}$ are *Long.* and *Circ.* strains, and $\{a_{lc}^{(i)}, a_{cl}^{(i)}\}$ are *Long.* - *Circ.* shearings. $\{a_{rl}^{(i)}, a_{rc}^{(i)}\}$ are *Rad.* displacement gradients in *Long.* and *Circ.* directions (not transmural). We then have 9×19 parameters for modeling the motion of each of the endo/mid/epi layers.

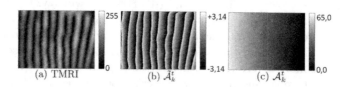

(a) TMRI   (b) $\tilde{\mathcal{A}}_k^t$ (c) $\mathcal{A}_k^t$

Fig. 1. Illustration of (a) the TMRI image, (b) the HARP phase, (c) the unwrapped phase computed taking a pixel's phase value as reference.

3.2   Phase-Based Registration *Without* Constraint

We aim to optimize the motion $\mathbf{v}$ according to phase-based SSD [6]:

$$E_{phase}(\mathbf{v}) = \int_\Omega \sum_{k=0}^{2} \omega_k(\mathbf{x}, \mathbf{u}(\mathbf{x}))\left(\mathcal{A}_k^{ref}(\mathbf{x}) - \mathcal{A}_k^t(\mathbf{x} + \mathbf{u}(\mathbf{x}) + \mathbf{v}(\mathbf{x}))\right)^2 d\mathbf{x} \quad (2)$$

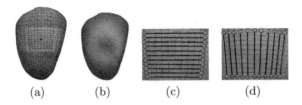

Fig. 2. The surface layer mesh with windows and the definition of control point pairs. (a): LV mesh and windows; (b): the window function $\varphi^{(i)}(\mathbf{x})$; (c), (d) show respectively the control point pairs in *Circ.* and *Long.* directions.

Where k indicates the sequence, and ref indicates the reference time (the last frame in our case). $\mathcal{A}_k^t$ is the unwrapped phase as is illustrated in Fig. 1. We use the unwrapped phase for the formulation because it facilitates the computation of tag numbers which will be described later in Sect. 3.3. Both $\mathbf{u}$ and $\mathbf{v}$ are motions from ref to t. $\mathbf{u}$ is the current motion which is known, while $\mathbf{v}$ is the motion model in Eq. 1. We opt for registering all other frames to ref for avoiding the accumulation of errors during the tracking. ω_k is a weight function introduced in [6]. The reader is referred to [6] for more details.

3.3   Phase-Based Registration *With* Constraint

In this section, we describe how to implement the NTC for refining the motion. It is rather intuitive that the number of tags between two material points remains unchanged throughout the cardiac cycle. As a consequence, we propose to add an additional constraint energy to Eq. 2 for penalizing the deviation of tag numbers to that at ref.

First, we select a number of myocardial point pairs following the *circ.* and *long.* directions as shown in Fig. 2(c) and (d). For each window, the boundary mesh nodes are paired in *circ.* and *long.* directions. Those node pairs are chosen for defining the constraint. We take all such point pairs from the mid-level and apical windows. Those from the basal windows are excluded because segmentation errors are more severe [1]. We denote these point pairs by $(\mathbf{p}_j, \mathbf{q}_j)$ with $j = 0$ to $J - 1$ where $\mathbf{p}_j$ and $\mathbf{q}_j$ are the material coordinates at ref time.

The number of tag between $\mathbf{p}_j$ and $\mathbf{q}_j$ is then computed by normalizing their unwrapped phase difference by 2π. The constraint energy is defined as follows:

$$E_c(\mathbf{v}) = \sum_{j=0}^{J-1} \sum_{k=0}^{2} \left(\frac{1}{2\pi} \mathcal{D}_{k,j}^{ref} - \frac{1}{2\pi} \mathcal{D}_{k,j}^t \right)^2$$

$$\text{with } \mathcal{D}_{k,j}^{ref} = \mathcal{A}_k^{ref}(\mathbf{q}_j) - \mathcal{A}_k^{ref}(\mathbf{p}_j) \tag{3}$$

$$\mathcal{D}_{k,j}^t = \mathcal{A}_k^t\big(\mathcal{T}_u(\mathbf{q}_j) + \mathbf{v}(\mathbf{q}_j)\big) - \mathcal{A}_k^t\big(\mathcal{T}_u(\mathbf{p}_j) + \mathbf{v}(\mathbf{p}_j)\big)$$

$$\mathcal{T}_u(\mathbf{x}) = \mathbf{x} + \mathbf{u}(\mathbf{x})$$

where $\mathbf{u}$ has the same definition as that in Eq. 2 and $\mathbf{v}$ is given by Eq. 1.

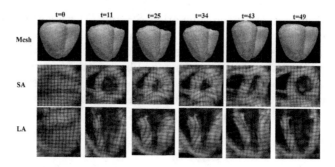

Fig. 3. Ground truth meshes, short- and long- axis slices of the synthetic TMRI (three sequences of line taggings are multiplied for better visualization).

E_c can be decomposed into a number of local quadratic forms. Actually, it is upper-bounded by the sum of those quadratic forms. The reader is referred to the appendix for more details on the derivation of the following equation:

$$E_c(\mathbf{v}) \leq \sum_i E_c^{(i)}(\mathbf{v}^{(i)}) \tag{4}$$

where i indicates the window, $\mathbf{v}^{(i)}$ is the local motion described in Eq. 1, and $E_c^{(i)}$ is the local quadratic form corresponding to the window i.

Similarly for $E_{phase}(\mathbf{v})$, we have $E_{phase}(\mathbf{v}) \leq \sum_i E_{phase}^{(i)}(\mathbf{v}^{(i)})$ with $E_{phase}^{(i)}$ being local quadratic forms according to [6]. Finally, by combining the phase-based term E_{phase} and the constraint energy E_c, we have E defined as:

$$E(\mathbf{v}) = E_{phase}(\mathbf{v}) + \lambda\xi E_c(\mathbf{v}) \leq \sum_i \left(E_{phase}^{(i)}(\mathbf{v}^{(i)}) + \lambda\xi E_c^{(i)}(\mathbf{v}^{(i)}) \right) \tag{5}$$

Where ξ is a normalizing factor. We set it to 10^3 empirically in our experiments. λ is the weight of the constraint. It is tuned later in Sect. 5.1. Equation 5 means that E is upbounded by the sum of local energies $E_{phase}^{(i)} + \lambda\xi E_c^{(i)}$. E is minimized by optimizing each of the local quadratic form through solving a linear system. The whole process is iterated until convergence.

4   Generation of Synthetic Images

We combined a real 3D TMRI recording denoted as $\mathcal{I}_k^t$ and an electro-mechanical (E/M) model simulating the cardiac electrophysiological activation and the myocardial contraction [8] for generating synthetic images.

It consists of four steps: (1) we track the LV in the real recording by [1]. The output is a sequence of volumetric meshes denoted as $\mathcal{M}^t$; (2) we use the E/M model to simulate myocardial deformations corresponding to the LV geometry $\mathcal{M}^0$, leading to another sequence of meshes $\mathcal{S}^t$; (3) since $\mathcal{M}^0$ and $\mathcal{S}^0$ are equivalent, it is easy to build a Thin Plate Spline (TPS) transformation that warps the real images $\mathcal{I}_k^t$ to the simulation $\mathcal{S}^t$; and (4) we correct the apparent motion extracted in (1) by transformations contained in $\mathcal{S}^t$ sequence so that the motion in the simulated images corresponds to the E/M model. Each myocardial voxel position at time t is mapped back to the first frame. The new intensity is then computed by linearly interpolating $\mathcal{I}_k^0$. In this study, we simulated a synthetic data for a normal heart shown in Fig. 3. The spatial resolution is $0.96 \times 0.96 \times 7.71\, mm$ and line tag spacing is $7\, mm$.

5   Result

5.1   Synthetic Data

We use the synthetic data for tuning the constraint weight λ (Eq. 5) and investigating whether the constraint helps improving strain accuracy. Here the evaluation only involves the mid layer where the constraint was used. We display in Fig. 4(a) the evolution of RMSE motion errors at end-systole with λ. From the result, we observe that there is an optimal value around $\lambda = 1.5$. We then compared the performance between using $\lambda = 0$ and $\lambda = 1.5$ on strain quantification in Fig. 4(b) and (c). We used the Engineering strain as described in [1]. We see that for both strains, using the constraint gives smaller RMSE strain errors. This confirms the interest of utilizing the NTC constraint.

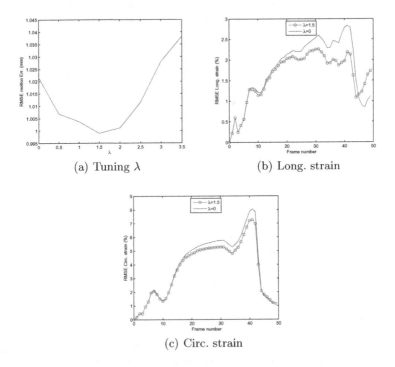

(a) Tuning λ (b) Long. strain

(c) Circ. strain

Fig. 4. (a):Evolution of motion errors at end-systole with the constraint energy weight λ; (b): Temporal evolution of Long. and (c): Circ. strain errors.

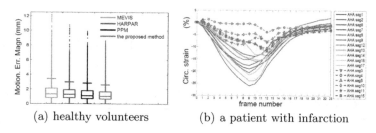

(a) healthy volunteers   (b) a patient with infarction

Fig. 5. (a): Volunteer data landmark tracking errors using $\lambda = 1.5$ compared to the state-of-the-art; (b) Circ. strain curves on a patient with fibrosis. Solid lines show normal segments while curves with markers show segments with fibrosis.

5.2 Real Data

We also evaluated our method on 15 healthy volunteer datasets which are publicly available from [9]. Each volunteer data has 24 manually tracked landmarks located in the basal, mid and apical myocardium. These landmarks were warped forward in time by computing barycentric coordinates in the first frame and propagating them through the sequence of volumetric meshes. From Fig. 5(a), we see that the dispersion of motion errors is reduced when compared to the purely phase-based registration (without NTC constraint) PPM [6]. This result is further confirmed by Levene's test. The returned p-value is below 0.05, rejecting the null hypothesis that their variances are equal. Besides, our method slightly outperformed the other two recent methods HARPAR (regularized HARP) [1] and MEVIS (quadrature-filter based) [9] in both median and variance values.

Moreover, our method was evaluated on a patient who had fibrosis at the entire inferior wall, part of the inferolateral wall and part of the inferoseptal wall (AHA n° 3,4,5,10,11,15) confirmed by late-enhancement MR. In Fig. 5(b) we observe reduced *Circ.* strain values for those infarcted segments, showing a clear discrepancy between normal segments and those with fibrosis.

6   Conclusion and Discussion

This paper integrates the NTC constraints into a recent phase-based registration framework for refining the tracking. On synthetic data, we observe that integrating the constraint improved both motion and strain (*Long.* and *Circ.*) accuracies. On healthy volunteers, the proposed method gives better accuracy compared to three state-of-the-art algorithms. On a patient with infarction, we observe reduced *Circ.*strain values for those AHA segments with fibrosis. We admit that a more thorough validation needs to be done both synthetically and clinically in the future. However, our aim is to show the potential benefits of combining respective advantages of both methods (tracking-based and Gabor-based non-tracking), which we consider as an interesting research field.

Appendix

In Eq. 3, conducting 1st-order approximations on $\mathcal{A}_k^t$ leads to:

$$E_c(\mathbf{v}) \approx$$
$$\sum_j \sum_k \left(\frac{\mathcal{A}_k^{ref}(\mathbf{q}_j) - \mathcal{A}_k^{ref}(\mathbf{p}_j)}{2\pi} - \frac{\mathcal{A}_k^t(\mathcal{T}_u(\mathbf{q}_j)) - \mathcal{A}_k^t(\mathcal{T}_u(\mathbf{p}_j)) + \delta_k^j(\mathbf{v})}{2\pi} \right)^2 \quad (6)$$

with $\delta_k^j(\mathbf{v}) = \nabla \mathcal{A}_k^t(\mathcal{T}_u(\mathbf{q}_j)) \cdot \mathbf{v}(\mathbf{q}_j) - \nabla \mathcal{A}_k^t(\mathcal{T}_u(\mathbf{p}_j)) \cdot \mathbf{v}(\mathbf{p}_j)$

Instead of computing $\mathcal{A}_k^t$ maps by phase unwrapping which is highly sensitive to image artifacts, we chose to circumvent the issue by (1) computing $\nabla \mathcal{A}_k^t$ from HARP phases by the method described in [2] and (2) further computing $\mathcal{A}_k^\tau(\mathbf{q}_j) - \mathcal{A}_k^\tau(\mathbf{p}_j)$ ($\tau = ref$ and t) by curvilinear integration of $\nabla \mathcal{A}_k^\tau$. The path of integration is easily defined using our mesh topology. Equation 6 then becomes:

$$E_c(\mathbf{v}) = \sum_j \sum_k \left(\beta_k^j - \frac{1}{2\pi} \delta_k^j(\mathbf{v}) \right)^2$$
$$\text{with } \beta_k^j = \frac{1}{2\pi} \int_{\mathbf{p}_j}^{\mathbf{q}_j} \nabla \mathcal{A}_k^{ref}(\mathbf{x}) d\mathbf{x} - \frac{1}{2\pi} \int_{\mathcal{T}_u(\mathbf{p}_j)}^{\mathcal{T}_u(\mathbf{q}_j)} \nabla \mathcal{A}_k^t(\mathbf{x}) d\mathbf{x} \quad (7)$$

where β_k^j is known and $\delta_k^j(\mathbf{v})$ contains the model parameters.

We first replace both $\varphi^{(i)}(\mathbf{p}_j)$ and $\varphi^{(i)}(\mathbf{q}_j)$ in $\delta_k^j(\mathbf{v})$ by $g_j^{(i)} = \frac{\varphi^{(i)}(\mathbf{p}_j) + \varphi^{(i)}(\mathbf{q}_j)}{2}$. This is justified by the fact that $\mathbf{p}_j$ and $\mathbf{q}_j$ are symmetric to the window center (see Fig. 2), thus $\varphi^{(i)}(\mathbf{p}_j) \approx \varphi^{(i)}(\mathbf{q}_j)$. $\delta_k^j(\mathbf{v})$ then becomes:

$$\delta_k^j(\mathbf{v}) \approx \sum_i g_j^{(i)} \mathcal{L}_j^{(i)}(\mathbf{v}^{(i)})$$
$$\text{with } \mathcal{L}_j^{(i)}(\mathbf{v}^{(i)}) = \nabla \mathcal{A}_k^t(\mathcal{T}_u(\mathbf{q}_j)) \cdot \mathbf{v}^{(i)}(\mathbf{q}_j) - \nabla \mathcal{A}_k^t(\mathcal{T}_u(\mathbf{p}_j)) \cdot \mathbf{v}^{(i)}(\mathbf{p}_j) \quad (8)$$

Then, applying the *Partition-of-Unity* property [7] of $g_j^{(i)}$ leads directly to [7]:

$$E_c(\mathbf{v}) \leq \sum_i \sum_j g_j^{(i)} \sum_k \left(\beta_k^j - \frac{1}{2\pi} \mathcal{L}_j^{(i)}(\mathbf{v}^{(i)}) \right)^2 = \sum_i E_c^{(i)}(\mathbf{v}^{(i)}) \quad (9)$$

Where $E_c^{(i)}$ is quadratic since $\mathcal{L}_j^{(i)}$ is linear in the motion parameters of $\mathbf{v}^{(i)}$.

References

1. Zhou, Y., Bernard, O., Saloux, E., Manrique, A., Allain, P., Makram-Ebeid, S., De Craene, M.: 3D harmonic phase tracking with anatomical regularization. Med. Image Anal. **26**(1), 70–81 (2015)

2. Osman, N.F., Kerwin, W.S., McVeigh, E.R., Prince, J.L.: Cardiac motion tracking using cine harmonic phase (HARP) magnetic resonance imaging. Magn. Reson. Med. **42**(6), 1048 (1999)
3. Qian, Z., Liu, Q., Metaxas, D.N., Axel, L.: Identifying regional cardiac abnormalities from myocardial strains using nontracking-based strain estimation and spatiotemporal tensor analysis. IEEE Trans. Med. Imaging **30**(12), 2017–2029 (2011)
4. Bruurmijn, L.C.M., Kause, H.B., Filatova, O.G., Duits, R., Fuster, A., Florack, L.M.J., Assen, H.C.: Myocardial deformation from local frequency estimation in tagging MRI. In: Ourselin, S., Rueckert, D., Smith, N. (eds.) FIMH 2013. LNCS, vol. 7945, pp. 284–291. Springer, Heidelberg (2013). doi:10.1007/978-3-642-38899-6_34
5. Kause, H.B., Filatova, O.G., Duits, R., Bruurmijn, L.C.M., Fuster, A., Westenberg, J.J.M., Florack, L.M.J., van Assen, H.C.: Direct myocardial strain assessment from frequency estimation in tagging MRI. In: Camara, O., Mansi, T., Pop, M., Rhode, K., Sermesant, M., Young, A. (eds.) STACOM 2013. LNCS, vol. 8330, pp. 212–219. Springer, Heidelberg (2014). doi:10.1007/978-3-642-54268-8_25
6. Zhou, Y., De Craene, M., Bernard, O.: Phase-based registration of cardiac tagged mr images using anatomical deformation model. In: 2016 IEEE 13th International Symposium on Biomedical Imaging (ISBI), pp. 617–620. IEEE (2016)
7. Makram-Ebeid, S., Somphone, O.: Non-rigid image registration using a hierarchical partition of unity finite element method. In: 2007 IEEE 11th International Conference on Computer Vision ICCV 2007, pp. 1–8. IEEE (2007)
8. Marchesseau, S., Delingette, H., Sermesant, M., Ayache, N.: Fast parameter calibration of a cardiac electromechanical model from medical images based on the unscented transform. Biomech. Model. Mechanobiol. **12**(4), 815–831 (2013)
9. Tobon-Gomez, C., De Craene, M., Mcleod, K., Tautz, L., Shi, W., Hennemuth, A., Prakosa, A., Wang, H., Carr-White, G., Kapetanakis, S., et al.: Benchmarking framework for myocardial tracking and deformation algorithms: An open access database. Med. Image Anal. **17**(6), 632–648 (2013)

Segmentation and Registration Coupling from Short-Axis Cine MRI: Application to Infarct Diagnosis

Stephanie Marchesseau[1($\boxtimes$)], Nicolas Duchateau[2], and Hervé Delingette[2]

[1] Clinical Imaging Research Centre, A*STAR-NUS, Singapore, Singapore
stephanie_marchesseau@nuhs.edu.sg
[2] Asclepios Research Project, Inria Sophia Antipolis, Valbonne, France

Abstract. Estimating regional deformation of the myocardium from Cine MRI has the potential to locate abnormal tissue. Regional deformation of the left ventricle is commonly estimated using either segmentation or $3D + t$ registration. Segmentation is often performed at each instant separately from the others. It can be tedious and does not guarantee temporal causality. On the other hand, extracting regional parameters through image registration is highly dependent on the initial segmentation chosen to propagate the deformation fields and may not be consistent with the myocardial contours. In this paper, we propose an intermediate approach that couples segmentation and registration in order to improve temporal causality while removing the influence of the chosen initial segmentation. We propose to apply the deformation fields from image registration (sparse Bayesian registration) to every segmentation of the cardiac cycle and combine them for more robust regional measurements. As an illustration, we describe local deformation through the measurement of AHA regional volumes. Maximum regional volume change is extracted and compared across scar and non-scar regions defined from delayed enhancement MRI on 20 ST-elevation myocardial infarction patients. The proposed approach shows (i) more robustness in extracting regional volumes than direct segmentation or standard registration and (ii) better performance in detecting scar.

Keywords: Regional volumes · Segmentation · Registration · Infarct diagnosis

1 Introduction

Local tracking of the myocardium has shown to help determining the local viability of the heart from MRI [10] or echocardiography [4]. Two ways to measure regional deformation are reported in most papers: (i) the sequence of 3D segmentations (named here *Segmentation*) and (ii) the sequence made of an initial 3D geometry propagated in time using the output of the image registration along the sequence (named here *3D segmentation + registration*). Manual

© Springer International Publishing AG 2017
T. Mansi et al. (Eds.): STACOM 2016, LNCS 10124, pp. 48–56, 2017.
DOI: 10.1007/978-3-319-52718-5_6

or semi-automatic segmentation as offered in commercial software is straight-forward, does not rely on any hypothesis from a registration algorithm and is usually considered as ground truth. However, it is a fastidious process leading to variable results between observers, non-consistency between slices or frames and requiring several manual adjustments. To tackle this issue, many research groups have worked on automatic segmentation [11], with some recent methods that include spatio-temporal information to propagate the segmentation [7,13]. Despite these progresses, routine delineation of the ventricles is still semi-automatic, which offers more confidence and flexibility to the cardiologists. 3D segmentation + registration, on the other hand, gives smooth results in space and time and better consistency between frames. However, full temporal consistency is still not guaranteed and the method can be inconsistent with the myocardial contours (Fig. 1 left). Moreover, standard 3D segmentation + registration heavily depends on the first 3D segmentation used to propagate the deformation fields (Fig. 1 right) leading to high uncertainty on the quantification of the deformation. The dependence on the frame selection and the temporal consistency issue have already been considered in the design of registration algorithms, for instance on 3D echocardiographic data [3,12], although the segmentation from a single instant is considered.

We suggest to combine both the segmentation (of all time frames) and an independent registration algorithm by averaging the propagated mesh from every frame (and not only the first frame) in order to leverage the drawbacks of both while maintaining their assets. This approach is simple, registration-independent, and could be directly translated to clinical practice using already available segmentation software and image registration algorithms. Using this approach reduces the need for a temporally consistent segmentation or registration, since all frames of the cardiac cycle are used to propagate the registration output.

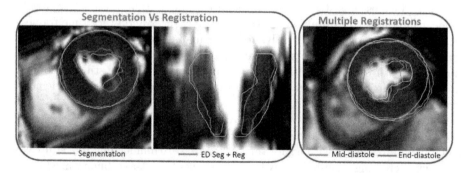

Fig. 1. (Left) Segmentation (green contours) compared to registration (purple contours) on short-axis and long-axis view. (Right) Comparison between segmentation (pink contours), the registration propagated from end-diastole (green contours) and the registration propagated from mid-diastole (frame 20, blue contours), for a mid-systole short-axis slice. (Color figure online)

The ultimate goal of registration or segmentation is to extract quantitative parameters in order to understand, estimate, and classify patient's motion, deformation or shape abnormalities. As an application, we intend to detect abnormal AHA zones from regional volume changes using the standard two approaches and our proposed coupling method. Regional volumes are clinical indices already measured in clinical practice from echocardiography [2] in some cases but rarely measured in MRI partly due to insufficient reliability of the current methods. Previous work also used regional volumes as a way to personalise an electro-mechanical model as it overcomes the aperture problem of tracking contours using Cine MRI only [9].

2   Methods

2.1   Patient Population and Pre-processing

Image Acquisition. To validate the proposed method against alternatives, 20 patient scans were collected from 3 different clinical studies. The first 10 patients were recruited after ST-elevation myocardial infarction and images were acquired on a Siemens 3 T mMR. The next 10 patients were scanned on a Philips 3T Ingenia after ST-elevation myocardial infarction. Ethical approval and written consent were obtained for all patients. Imaging protocol consisted of 2 chambers, 3 chambers, 4 chambers and short-axis stack Cine images to evaluate the cardiac function as well as short-axis delayed enhancement (LGE) sequences 10 min after injection of 0.4 mmol/kg of Gadolinium. Image resolution varied between $1.32 \times 1.32 \times 9\,\text{mm}^3$ and $1.42 \times 1.42 \times 10\,\text{mm}^3$ and contained 25 to 30 frames per cardiac cycle.

Short-axis image processing. All images were analyzed by 3 experts on Segment[1] and then manually corrected after consensus. Image processing of the Cine MRI images consisted of semi-automatic segmentation of the left ventricle endocardium and epicardium on all the short-axis slices and every time frames. Image processing of the LGE MRI required manual segmentation of the left ventricle and semi-automatic segmentation of the scar using Otsu thresholding model [5], as thresholding methods and manual corrections are still the clinical standard despite progress [1,6] towards automatic infarct delineation as demonstrated in the STACOM'12 challenge.

3D modelling. MR spatial resolution of both the Cine and the LGE sequences is highly heterogeneous with a slice thickness of 9 to 10 mm leading to a staircase effect when creating a mesh directly from the stack of short-axis binary masks. To smooth this effect, the short-axis 2D segmentations were first realigned around the long-axis to prevent from potential artifacts due to to different breath holding positions. For this, the long-axis was defined as the line linking the barycentres of the apical and basal endocardial contours. For each slice, the barycentre of

---

[1] Segment is a freely available software available at http://segment.heiberg.se.

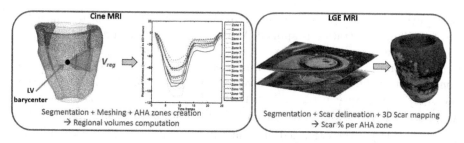

Fig. 2. (Left) Division of the 3D mesh into AHA zones for the creation of regional volumes defined as the volume between the barycentre of the LV and the endocardial surface of the AHA zone. (Right) 3D mapping of the scar regions from short-axis LGE images.

the endocardium was then translated to the long-axis. Second, the polygons formed by each 2D binary masks were linearly interpolated in the z dimension to allow homogeneous resolution. 3D meshes were then created using the CGAL 4.8 library[2]. A sequence of 3D segmentations was therefore obtained from Cine MRI. From LGE images, a 3D geometry was created similarly from the endocardium and epicardium delineation. The 2D binary masks of scar delineation were then mapped onto this mesh after iso-resampling. 3D meshes were divided into 17 AHA zones and regional volumes for Cine MRI and scar percentage (number of mesh elements with a scar over the total size of the AHA zone) for LGE MRI, were computed for each AHA zone. Each AHA zone containing at least 1% scarred tissue was labeled as a scar zone. Figure 2 illustrates these two pipelines. The effect of spatial interpolation errors was minimized by averaging the measurements over the AHA zones, larger than the slice resolution.

2.2   Proposed Segmentation and Registration Coupling

Evaluation of local properties such as regional volume change, is usually performed by studying a time sequence of meshes created by segmentation or by propagation of deformation fields on an initial mesh. An intermediate approach that takes the advantages of both approaches is presented here.

Sparse Bayesian Registration. Image registration was based on the sparse Bayesian algorithm presented in [8]. Images were first upsampled to an isotropic resolution using a linear interpolator. Pairs of consecutive images are registered and the estimated transformations are chained along the cycle. Our implementation uses a three-level multiresolution scheme and the parameters described in [8], which were evaluated on the STACOM'11 registration challenge dataset.

Coupling segmentation and registration. In order to soften the heavy influence of the segmentation on the results of a registration, all 3D segmentations

---

[2] The Computational Geometry Algorithms Library is available at www.cgal.org.

of the cardiac cycle are used in our approach as an initial mesh to which the corresponding registration is applied. More precisely, let's call M_t the mesh created from the segmentation of the cardiac frame t and $f_{j \to j+1}$ the deformation field computed from the registration of frames j to $j+1$. These deformation fields may be composed and inverted to register any frame into another one: $f_{i \to j} = f_{i \to k} \circ \cdots \circ f_{j-1 \to j}$. Therefore, if the cardiac cycle is imaged into N frames, there exists N possible meshes for each frame: $\{M_i^j\}_{i \in [1,N]}$ where $M_i^j = f_{i \to j}(M_i)$ is the deformed mesh at time j coming from the segmentation of frame i.

2.3   Regional Volumes

In this paper we decided to focus on regional volume changes as an index for local contraction deficiency caused by the presence of scar tissue (as previously shown using a electromechanical model of the heart in [9]). Regional volumes are defined as the volume formed by the endocardial surface of the AHA zone and the barycentre of the LV (Fig. 2 left). This measure is segmentation-based and can be easily measured from independent meshes. Additionally, this measure is robust to small registration or segmentation errors since it averages the displacements of all points of the selected surface. We compute it via three different ways:

(i) **Segmentation:** Regional volumes are computed for each mesh created directly from the segmentation and compiled as a time sequence for each AHA zone α:

$$V_{reg_\alpha}^{Seg}(j) = V_{reg_\alpha}(M_j)$$

(ii) **3D segmentation + registration:** AHA zones are created on the end-diastolic mesh and this mesh is deformed under the registration deformation fields. Consistent regional volumes sequences are then extracted for each zone:

$$V_{reg_\alpha}^{3DSeg+Reg}(j) = V_{reg_\alpha}(f_{0 \to j}(M_0))$$

(iii) **Our coupling: segmentation + registration:** Regional volumes are computed for every combination of 3D segmentation + registration and the mean value measured for each time point:

$$V_{reg_\alpha}^{Coupling}(j) = \frac{1}{N} \sum_{i=0}^{N} V_{reg_\alpha}(f_{i \to j}(M_i))$$

2.4   Statistical Analysis

We hypothesize that maximum regional volume change enables to detect zones containing scar tissue. Regional volume changes were computed as the relative difference between the regional volume at time t and the regional volume at time 0 (end-diastole). The maximum regional volume change was then measured as the minimum over time of the regional volume change (also called regional ejection fraction). Maximum regional volume change of scar and healthy zones were compared statistically using Student's t-test and the level of statistical significance was set to a p-value < 0.05. Additionally, in order to evaluate the accuracy of the regional volumes in predicting the position of a scar zone, ROC analysis was performed and the Area Under Curve (AUC) computed. A perfect prediction tool corresponds to an AUC of 1 while a AUC of 0.5 corresponds to a coin toss.

3   Results

3.1   Comparison of Volume Changes Between Methods

Differences in the application of the deformation fields from the end-diastolic frame or any other frame were noticed for every case. Figure 3 (bottom) illustrates three examples on the same patient where the propagation from the first frame (red contours), the segmentation (green contours), and the coupling curve (blue contours), lead to different contraction levels. These differences impact the computation of the regional volumes (Fig. 3 top). The left column illustrates ideal cases where all three methods agree with a small difference. The middle column illustrates examples where the segmentation is unreliable and inconsistent in time leading to noisy regional volumes, probably due to inclusion/exclusion of papillary muscles as shown in the bottom row. For these cases, using a registration algorithm enables to smooth the results and improve the temporal consistency,

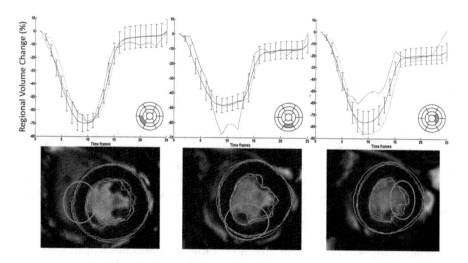

Fig. 3. (Top) Examples of regional volume change (between each frame and the first frame, leading to a change of 0% at time 0 for all methods) of 1 patient, for 3 AHA zones: (red) 3D Segmentation + registration, (green) segmentation, (blue) distribution over the set of segmentations where the mean is the selected value for our coupling approach. (Bottom) Corresponding short-axis images where yellow circles highlight the AHA zone to consider. Contours are colored with the same code as the above curves. (Color figure online)

for both the standard registration or the proposed coupling. For the right column, both the standard approaches are incorrect: the segmentation is noisy but within an acceptable level, however the registration using the first frame leads to overestimated contraction. The standard deviation of volume changes over all the segmentations propagated to a given frame is represented by a blue errorbar. Its average amplitude at end-systole around 20% illustrates the high influence of the initial mesh for the quantification of the deformation.

3.2   Ability to Locate Scar Zones

As shown in Fig. 4, all methods agree that maximum regional volume change is lower for scar zones (in red) than for healthy tissue (in blue) for every AHA zone. This difference is even significant ($p < 0.05$) for 7 or 6 of the 17 AHA zones depending on the method used to calculate the regional volumes. Note that lateral zones (5, 6, 11, 12) present only 0 to 3 scar regions making statistical significance unreachable. It is also interesting to note that the mean healthy regional volume is highly dependent on the AHA zone. A unique threshold for the full myocardium would therefore be inadequate.

More precisely, segmentation seems to be the least reliable of the three methods and fails to differentiate the scars on zones 1 and 16. Moreover, 3D segmentation + registration fails to separate healthy from scar tissue on zone 11. Our coupling approach, on the other hand always differentiates scar vs non-scar regional volume changes.

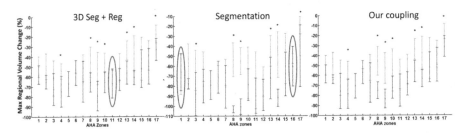

Fig. 4. Maximum regional volume changes for each AHA zones using the 3 methods. Blue (resp. red) bars represent the means and standard deviations for healthy (resp. scar) areas. Stars (*) indicates significant differences ($p < 0.05$). Green ellipses highlight failed differentiation. (Color figure online)

Additionally, AUC values are presented Table 1 and examples of ROC curves that led to the measurements of AUC values are shown Fig. 5. The mean accuracy of the coupling method (0.84 ± 0.10) is significantly higher than the standard segmentation method (0.78 ± 0.14) and higher than the standard 3D segmentation + registration approach (0.82 ± 0.10) although not significantly. Additionally, the coupling methods reaches the best detection in 8 zones. In contrast, segmentation is better than our coupling in 5 zones and 3D segmentation + registration in 3 zones. Finally, the proposed approach never shows the worst performance.

Table 1. AUC (Area under Curve) values from ROC analysis for each AHA zone and each method for the accuracy in the detection of the scar zone. Bold values represent best accuracy.

AHA zone	1	2	3	4	5	6	7	8	9	10	11	12	13	14	15	16	17
n. of scars	9	17	12	3	0	1	13	17	13	4	2	3	15	17	8	5	15
4D Seg	0.56	0.76	**0.77**	0.82	0.00	**0.74**	0.68	**1.00**	1.00	0.63	0.78	0.75	0.85	**0.96**	**0.72**	0.61	0.87
Our coupling	**0.75**	**0.96**	0.73	0.90	0.00	0.63	**0.76**	**1.00**	0.96	0.75	**0.81**	0.76	0.96	0.92	0.67	**0.73**	0.88
3D Seg + Reg	0.74	0.88	0.71	**0.92**	0.00	0.53	0.71	0.86	0.89	**0.92**	0.78	0.75	**0.96**	0.92	0.66	0.72	**0.89**

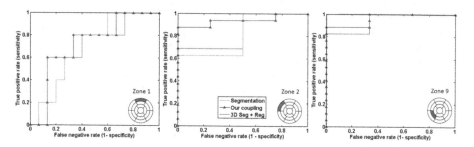

Fig. 5. Examples of ROC curves measuring the accuracy of the infarct detection for each 3 methods on 3 AHA zones.

4 Discussion and Conclusion

In this paper, we highlighted the lack of consistency between the two standard approaches for deformation estimation and the need for a more robust, intermediate approach. We proposed a coupling method that combines both the output of the registration and the segmentation of all the cardiac frames. We illustrated this method by measuring the regional volumes and studied their ability to detect infarct tissue on 20 patients. Results showed that segmentation, standard registration and our approach can all be accurate in the scar detection. However, the detection was more systematic using the proposed coupling, which gathers the best assets of both methods (ground truth segmentation, spacial and temporal smoothness) without their drawbacks (noisy segmentation, exclusion/inclusion of papillary muscles, influence of the initial frame). Moreover, this method can easily be translated into clinical practice and applied routinely from already available segmentation and registration tools. A larger database would be required to validate these results and allow a more precise localization of the scars from regional volumes. Future work will investigate better fusion algorithms for a more robust coupling approach than the current simple averaging. We will also study the extension of this approach to tagged images for the evaluation of cardiac motion through radial, circumferential and longitudinal strains.

Acknowledgement. This work has been partially funded by the NMRC NUHS Centre Grant Medical Image Analysis Core (NMRC/CG/013/2013) and by the European Research Council (MedYMA ERC-AdG-2011-291080).

References

1. Albà, X., Figueras i Ventura, R.M., Lekadir, K., Frangi, A.F.: Healthy and scar myocardial tissue classification in DE-MRI. In: Camara, O., Mansi, T., Pop, M., Rhode, K., Sermesant, M., Young, A. (eds.) STACOM 2012. LNCS, vol. 7746, pp. 62–70. Springer, Heidelberg (2013). doi:10.1007/978-3-642-36961-2_8

2. Auger, D., Ducharme, A., Harel, F., Marcotte, F., Thibault, B., O'Meara, E.: Patient assessment for cardiac resynchronization therapy: past, present and future of imaging techniques. Can. J. Cardiol. **26**(1), 27–34 (2010)

3. De Craene, M., Piella, G., Camara, O., Duchateau, N., Silva, E., Doltra, A., et al.: Temporal diffeomorphic free-form deformation: application to motion and strain estimation from 3D echocardiography. Med. Image Anal. **16**(2), 427–450 (2012)

4. Duchateau, N., De Craene, M., Allain, P., Saloux, E., Sermesant, M.: Infarct localization from myocardial deformation: prediction and uncertainty quantification by regression from a low-dimensional space. IEEE Trans. Med. Imaging **35**(10), 2340–2352 (2016)

5. Heiberg, E., Engblom, H., Engvall, J., Hedström, E., Ugander, M., Arheden, H.: Semi-automatic quantification of myocardial infarction from delayed contrast enhanced magnetic resonance imaging. Scand. Cardiovasc. J. **39**(5), 267–275 (2005)

6. Karim, R., et al.: Infarct segmentation challenge on delayed enhancement MRI of the left ventricle. In: Camara, O., Mansi, T., Pop, M., Rhode, K., Sermesant, M., Young, A. (eds.) STACOM 2012. LNCS, vol. 7746, pp. 97–104. Springer, Heidelberg (2013). doi:10.1007/978-3-642-36961-2_12

7. Atehortúa Labrador, A.M., Zuluaga, M.A., Ourselin, S., Giraldo, D., Castro, E.R.: Automatic segmentation of 4D cardiac MR images for extraction of ventricular chambers using a spatio-temporal approach. In: SPIE Medical Imaging. International Society for Optics and Photonics (2016)

8. Folgoc, L., Delingette, H., Criminisi, A., Ayache, N.: Sparse bayesian registration. In: Golland, P., Hata, N., Barillot, C., Hornegger, J., Howe, R. (eds.) MICCAI 2014. LNCS, vol. 8673, pp. 235–242. Springer, Heidelberg (2014). doi:10.1007/978-3-319-10404-1_30

9. Marchesseau, S., Delingette, H., Sermesant, M., Cabrera-Lozoya, R., Tobon-Gomez, C., Moireau, P., et al.: Personalization of a cardiac electromechanical model using reduced order unscented Kalman filtering from regional volumes. Med. Image Anal. **17**(7), 816–829 (2013)

10. Medrano-Gracia, P., Suinesiaputra, A., Cowan, B., Bluemke, D., Frangi, A., Lee, D., Lima, J., Young, A.: An atlas for cardiac MRI regional wall motion and infarct scoring. In: Camara, O., Mansi, T., Pop, M., Rhode, K., Sermesant, M., Young, A. (eds.) STACOM 2012. LNCS, vol. 7746, pp. 188–197. Springer, Heidelberg (2013). doi:10.1007/978-3-642-36961-2_22

11. Petitjean, C., Dacher, J.N.: A review of segmentation methods in short axis cardiac MR images. Med. Image Anal. **15**(2), 169–184 (2011)

12. Zhang, Z., Ashraf, M., Sahn, D.J., Song, X.: Temporally diffeomorphic cardiac motion estimation from three-dimensional echocardiography by minimization of intensity consistency error. Med. Phys. **41**(5), 052902 (2014)

13. Zhuang, X., Rhode, K., Razavi, R., Hawkes, D., Ourselin, S.: A registration-based propagation framework for automatic whole heart segmentation of cardiac MRI. IEEE Trans. Med. Imaging **29**(9), 1612–1625 (2010)

Learning Optimal Spatial Scales for Cardiac Strain Analysis Using a Motion Atlas

Matthew Sinclair[1]([✉]), Devis Peressutti[1], Esther Puyol-Antón[1], Wenjia Bai[2],
David Nordsletten[1], Myrianthi Hadjicharalambous[1], Eric Kerfoot[1],
Tom Jackson[1], Simon Claridge[1], C. Aldo Rinaldi[1], Daniel Rueckert[2],
and Andrew P. King[1]

[1] Division of Imaging Sciences and Biomedical Engineering,
King's College London, London, UK
`matthew.sinclair@kcl.ac.uk`
[2] Biomedical Image Analysis Group, Imperial College London, London, UK

Abstract. Cardiac motion is inherently tied to the disease state of the heart, and as such can be used to identify the presence and extent of different cardiac pathologies. Abnormal cardiac motion can manifest at different spatial scales of the myocardium depending on the disease present. The importance of spatial scale in the analysis of cardiac motion has not previously been explicitly investigated. In this paper, a novel approach is presented for analysing myocardial strains at different spatial scales using a cardiac motion atlas to find the optimal scales for (1) predicting response to cardiac resynchronisation therapy and (2) identifying the presence of strict left bundle-branch block in a patient cohort of 34. Optimal spatial scales for the two applications were found to be 4% and 16% of left ventricular volume with accuracies of 84.8±8.4% and 81.3±12.6%, respectively, using a repeated, stratified cross-validation.

1 Introduction

Cardiac motion is driven by the underlying electromechanics and perfusion, and has been increasingly assessed to predict the state and extent of cardiac disease. The comparison of cardiac motion across subject cohorts has been facilitated in recent years by the development of statistical motion atlases. A motion atlas entails the normalisation of subjects' cardiac geometry and motion both spatially and over time. Motion atlases have been used to identify abnormal cardiac motion [6,7,13], to predict scar location in the left ventricle (LV) [8,14], and to parcellate the LV based on motion as an alternative to AHA segments [1].

The importance of spatial scale in the analysis of cardiac motion has not been extensively investigated, despite the importance of scale in cardiac structure and function. As an example, the branching structure of the coronary vasculature follows power law relationships [3], and vessel generation has been shown to follow a power law in relation to downstream myocardial volume [12,17]. Disease in the coronary circulation is also known to manifest at different scales, both in the large coronary arteries and also at the microvascular scale [5]. Disease in the

T. Mansi et al. (Eds.): STACOM 2016, LNCS 10124, pp. 57–65, 2017.
DOI: 10.1007/978-3-319-52718-5_7

coronary circulation at different vessel scales entails different manifestations of perfusion abnormalities affecting function. This suggests that abnormal cardiac motion may manifest at different spatial scales depending on the disease, and that by extension there may be a characteristic tissue spatial scale at which cardiac deformation may be most predictive for different applications.

In this paper we present a novel framework based on computing strain at different spatial scales in the LV. This framework incorporates the use of a motion atlas with dimensionality reduction using principal component analysis (PCA) and classification using linear discriminant analysis (LDA) to identify the unique scale at which cardiac strain is most strongly predictive of different clinical parameters. We analyse myocardial strain due to its intrinsic link to tissue contractility, and due to its increased use in the clinical literature for the assessment of regional cardiac function (eg. [9]). In this study we apply our framework to the assessment of cardiac deformation at different scales in a cohort of cardiac resynchronisation therapy (CRT) patients, as detailed below.

2   Methods and Materials

2.1   Clinical Data

CRT is used to treat patients with electro-mechanical dyssynchrony which diminishes systolic function and can result in heart failure. Current clinical selection criteria for patients to undergo CRT include a NYHA functional class of II to IV, a QRS duration $> 120\,ms$, and an LV ejection fraction (EF) $< 35\%$ [11]. Response to CRT is defined as a decrease in end-systolic volume $\geq 15\%$. Under the current criteria, approximately 30% of patients undergoing CRT are non-responders, and improving on these criteria is an active field of research [11]. One factor influencing CRT response is the presence of strict left bundle-branch block (LBBB), defined by a longer QRS duration ($\geq 140\,ms$ in men and $\geq 130\,ms$ in women) and a mid-QRS notching [19], and characterised by dyssynchronous contraction of the septum relative to the LV lateral wall. While LBBB has a characteristic large-scale motion abnormality, it is yet unknown whether there is a particular scale of cardiac motion that distinguishes CRT responders' hearts from those of non-responders. A cohort of 34 CRT patients was considered in this study. LBBB was identified in 23/34 patients pre-CRT, and at a 6 month follow-up 26/34 patients were determined to be responders to CRT. The classification tasks considered in this study (see Sect. 3) are the identification of LBBB and the prediction of CRT response. Note that the prediction of CRT response was performed prospectively, i.e. using pre-CRT imaging data.

All patients underwent MR imaging before CRT using a 1.5 T scanner (Achieva, Philips Healthcare, Best, Netherlands), with the acquisition of ECG-gated, breath-hold cine-MR and T-MR (3D-tagged) sequences. A single multi-slice short axis (SA) and three single-slice long axis (LA) cine-MR sequences were acquired. Slice thickness was $8\,mm$ and $10\,mm$ for SA and LA sequences respectively, with an in-plane resolution for both of $\approx 1.4\,mm$. Three orthogonal T-MR sequences were combined to produce a $3D + t$ image with $\approx 1.0\,mm$

isotropic resolution. The SA and LA cine-MR sequences were rigidly aligned to the T-MR coordinate system, compensating for motion occurring between sequential breath-holds. The T-MR sequence was chosen as reference as it was free from respiratory motion.

2.2   Spatio-Temporal Motion Atlas

A motion atlas of the LV was formed to allow comparison of motion between patients. This process was based on frameworks proposed in a number of previous works (e.g. [6,13]). The main novelty in this study is the computation of myocardial strains at different spatial scales from a deforming LV point-cloud, and the investigation of application-specific scales for subsequent analysis. A framework for this approach is shown in Fig. 1, with the steps therein detailed below.

(A) LV Geometry Definition. The LV myocardium was manually segmented in the end-diastolic (ED) SA stack and 3 LA slices, excluding papillary muscles. The segmentations from the SA and LA images were subsequently fused and manually smoothed at a $2\,mm$ isotropic resolution. Following the identification of anatomical landmarks, a statistical shape model (SSM) was optimised to fit to the endocardial and epicardial surfaces of the LV binary segmentation [2], providing point-correspondence between patient hearts. The overlap of the SSM with each patient's LV geometry was visually assessed and the above process refined if necessary to ensure suitable overlap for subsequent motion tracking. In order to reduce the number of vertices of the SSM surface mesh (≈ 22000), a medial surface with regularly sampled vertices (≈ 3000) was generated via a combination of ray-casting and homogeneous downsampling followed by cell subdivision. Point-correspondence was retained by applying the same approach to each patient based on the initial point-correspondence of the SSM.

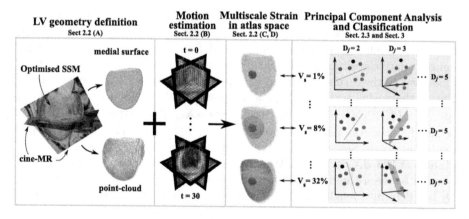

Fig. 1. An illustration of the proposed framework, with reference to relevant sections.

(B) Motion Tracking. The high resolution $3D + t$ T-MR sequence was then used for motion tracking. DICOM header information was used to determine the fraction of the cardiac cycle over which each $3D+t$ T-MR sequence was acquired, and temporal normalisation was performed for each patient, so that $t \in [0, 1)$, with 0 being ED and 1 being the end of the cardiac cycle. A $3D$ GPU-based B-spline free-form deformation (FFD) registration was used [16] to estimate LV motion between consecutive frames of the T-MR sequence. Subsequently, the inter-frame transformations were composed to estimate motion between each time frame and the ED time frame, producing a $3D + t$ B-spline transformation, ψ. In order to compare cardiac phases between patients, the reference ED medial surface was warped using ψ over $t \in [0, 1]$ at 30 equally spaced cardiac phases. The typical available fraction of the cardiac cycle from each T-MR sequence was 80%, so the first 24 frames of each transformation were used, $t \in [0, 0.8]$. The motion of each patient's LV was therefore fully represented by 24 deformed meshes.

(C) Multiscale Strain Calculation. In addition to producing a medial surface, the myocardial volume enclosed by the fitted SSM was sampled in a regular grid with half the resolution of the T-MR images (i.e. with an isotropic spacing of $\approx 2\,mm$). This produced point-clouds with ≈ 30000 points for each patient LV. The $3D + t$ motion transformation ψ was applied to the point-cloud to transform it to each of the cardiac phases at times, t, for each patient. At time $t=0$, at each point, i, on the medial surface, $P_{i,t=0}^{m}$, a neighbourhood of K nearest-neighbour points in the point-cloud, $\{P_{i,k,t=0}^{pc}\}, k = 1, \ldots, K$, were selected. These points were selected based on a percentage volume of the LV, representing a spatial scale. Six spatial scales were chosen following a power law, namely $V_s = 2^s\%, s \in [0, 1, 2, 3, 4, 5]$, (i.e. 1%, 2%, 4%, 8%, 16%, 32%) of the total LV volume, corresponding to approximately $K_s = 300 \times 2^s, s \in [0, 1, 2, 3, 4, 5]$ points in a neighbourhood at each respective scale. The method for computing strain at each $P_{i,t}^{m}$ from its deforming neighbourhood $\{P_{i,k,t}^{pc}\}, k = 1, \ldots, K$ is described below.

From large deformation mechanics, the deformation gradient tensor $\boldsymbol{F}$ maps the relative spatial position of two neighbouring particles before deformation $(d\boldsymbol{X})$ to their relative spatial position after deformation $(d\boldsymbol{x})$ [4]. The mapping from the relative position at the ED time frame $(d\boldsymbol{X})$ to that at every other time frame $(d\boldsymbol{x}_t)$ in the cardiac cycle can be expressed as $d\boldsymbol{x}_t = \boldsymbol{F}_t d\boldsymbol{X}$. Considering a point on the medial surface $P_{i,t=0}^{m}$ and its point-cloud neighbourhood at a given scale (s), $\{P_{i,k,t=0}^{pc}\}, k = 1, \ldots, K_s$, the vector $d\boldsymbol{X}_{i,k} \in \mathbb{R}^3$ expresses the $[x, y, z]$ distance between the pair of points $P_{i,t=0}^{m}$ and $P_{i,k,t=0}^{pc}$ at the undeformed ED time frame, $t = 0$. Stacking these vectors for all k neighbours gives a matrix of distances at ED, $d\hat{\boldsymbol{X}}_i \in \mathbb{R}^{K_s \times 3}$. At each consecutive time point, t, computing the distances between the deformed medial surface point $P_{i,t}^{m}$ and the same (as at ED) but deformed neighbours $\{P_{i,k,t}^{pc}\}, k = 1, \ldots, K_s$, we get the deformed distance matrices $d\hat{\boldsymbol{x}}_{i,t} \in \mathbb{R}^{K_s \times 3}$. The deformation gradient $\boldsymbol{F}_{i,t} \in \mathbb{R}^{3 \times 3}$ satisfying $d\hat{\boldsymbol{x}}_{i,t} = \boldsymbol{F}_{i,t} d\hat{\boldsymbol{X}}_i$ at medial surface point, i, and time, t, is then computed from the least-squares minimisation of $\sum_k \left\| d\hat{x}_{i,t} - F_{i,t} d\hat{X}_i \right\|^2$. Neighbourhood strain is computed using the Green-Lagrange strain tensor, $E_{i,t} = \frac{1}{2}(F_{i,t}{}^T F_{i,t} - I)$. For each patient, this computation was performed for every time frame, at every medial surface vertex and for neighbourhoods at each spatial scale V_s. Compute time for strain at all medial surface vertices for a given patient for a single frame ranged from approximately $3s$ at $V_0 = 1\%$ to $100s$ at $V_5 = 32\%$ on 8 CPUs.

(D) Spatial Normalisation. Differences in patient-specific LV geometries result in a biased comparison of motion between patients, which spatial normalisation is used to correct. Strains were reoriented from the patient-specific to the atlas coordinate space, similarly to how displacements [15] and velocities [6,7] have previously been reoriented. For each patient n, strain in atlas space, $E_{i,t,n}^{\text{atlas}}$, was computed via the Green-Lagrange strain tensor from the reoriented deformation tensor $F_{i,t,n}^{\text{atlas}} = J_{i,\phi_{n,t}} F_{i,t,n}^{\text{pat}} J_{i,\phi_{n,t}}^{-1}$, where $J_{i,\phi_{n,t}}$ is the Jacobian at time t of the patient-to-atlas transformation ϕ_n. Finally the reoriented strain $E_{i,t,n}^{\text{atlas}}$ was projected into a local atlas coordinate system in radial, r, longitudinal, l, and circumferential, c, directions. The main diagonal of the locally transported Green-Lagrange strain tensor provided the local strain components, $e_{i,t,n}^{\text{atlas}} = [e_{i,t,n}^{r}, e_{i,t,n}^{l}, e_{i,t,n}^{c}]$, for each patient, n, cardiac phase, t, and medial surface point, i, consistent with a clinically used coordinate system [9]. Figure 2 illustrates the scale-dependent strains (the mean of e^{atlas} at each vertex) at an end-systolic time frame for a patient with LBBB.

2.3   Dimensionality Reduction and Classification

The local strains in atlas space $e_{i,t,n}^{\text{atlas}}$ were concatenated into a single row vector such that for patient n, $\hat{e}_n \in \mathbb{R}^M$, where $M = (3 \times T \times N_m)$, T is the number of cardiac phases and N_m is the number of points in the atlas medial surface

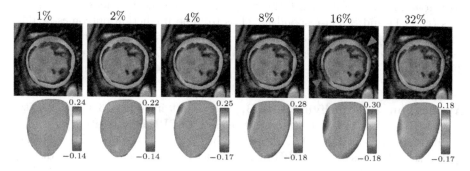

Fig. 2. Mean local strain displayed at different spatial scales on the LV medial surface at end-systole for a patient with LBBB (and septal flash), in a SA view (top) and a posterior LA view (bottom). Positive strains (stretching) are observed more distinctly in the septal region (red arrow) and negative strains (compression) are observed in the LV lateral wall (blue arrow), most strongly at $V_s = 16\%$ (Color figure online).

mesh. The row vector for each patient was then stacked to produce a matrix $X = \left[\hat{e}_1^T, \cdots, \hat{e}_{N_p}^T\right]^T \in \mathbb{R}^{N_p \times M}$, where N_p =number of patients. PCA was used to reduce the dimensionality of X to form $\tilde{X} \in \mathbb{R}^{N_p \times D}$ ($D \ll M$). LDA was used to classify patients from this low dimensional embedding $\tilde{X}$. Different numbers of PCA dimensions, D_j, were considered in the analysis.

In order to quantify accuracy as well as its standard deviation (SD) from this dataset, a repeated, stratified cross-validation (RSCV) was performed on $\tilde{X}_{j,s} \in \mathbb{R}^{N \times D_j}$, for each scale V_s and number of dimensions D_j. This involved dividing $\tilde{X}_{j,s}$ into training and validation data by randomly sampling from $\tilde{X}_{j,s}$ without replacement, while ensuring balanced classes in both training and validation datasets ('stratified'), and repeating this process to obtain a range of accuracy values at each D_j and V_s. A stratified approach to sampling was used since there are imbalanced classes in the data for the classification tasks.

3   Experiments and Results

A $\approx 75/25$ split was deemed suitable for the training data $\tilde{X}_{j,s}^{\text{train}}$ (26/34 patients) and validation data $\tilde{X}_{j,s}^{\text{val}}$ (8/34 patients), to allow for at least 2 observations from the smallest class (CRT non-responders, 8/34) to be represented in the validation set of each RSCV repetition. Experiments showed that accuracies and SDs stabilised after around 100 repetitions of the RSCV, which has been used for all results below. The optimal scale and number of dimensions for prediction of CRT response and identification of LBBB was selected as the combination of V_s and D_j that maximised the classification accuracy from the RSCV. Given the small size of the patient cohort (34 subjects), only up to the first 5 PCA dimensions were assessed to avoid over-fitting, specifically $D_j \in [2, 3, 4, 5]$. Accuracies, sensitivities and specificities are visualised in grids with respect to V_s (y-axis) and D_j (x-axis), as shown in Fig. 3.

Application 1: Predicting CRT response. The cohort included 26 responders (class 1) and 8 non-responders (class 0). The prediction outcomes at different values of D_j and V_s are shown in Fig. 3 (top row). The optimal spatial scale for predicting CRT response was $V_s = 4\%$ at $D_j = 2$, producing a prediction accuracy = $84.8 \pm 8.4\%$ (1SD), sensitivity = $94.0 \pm 8.1\%$ and specificity = $52.5 \pm 34.2\%$.

Application 2: Identifying LBBB. The cohort included 23 patients with strict LBBB (class 1) and 11 without it (class 0). LBBB identification outcomes at different values of D_j and V_s are shown in Fig. 3 (bottom row). The optimal spatial scale for classifying LBBB presence was $V_s = 16\%$ at $D_j = 3$, producing an accuracy = $81.3 \pm 12.6\%$, sensitivity = $90.2 \pm 12.9\%$ and specificity = $63.7 \pm 25.9\%$. This large spatial scale shows correspondence to the strong signal at 16% in the ED medial surface strain maps in Fig. 2.

4   Discussion

We have proposed a novel method for analysing strain at different spatial scales in the LV to identify an optimal scale for the classification of clinical parameters. Myocardial strain has not previously been analysed in the context of a motion atlas, nor has it been applied to the prediction of CRT response in the literature to the authors' knowledge. The accuracy achieved with our approach is comparable with the current state-of-the-art, where a volume-change systolic dyssynchrony index reported in [18] produced 85% sensitivity and 82% specificity. A 76% sensitivity and 100% specificity was reported in [10] by identifying a type II activation pattern.

Our results reveal that CRT response and LBBB are best predicted and identified, respectively, at different spatial scales. The larger optimal spatial scale of 16% for LBBB identification is consistent with the expected motion abnormality, i.e. septal flash. Figure 2 also illustrates that at end-systole, for a patient with LBBB, a visibly distinct difference in strains in the LV free wall and the septum

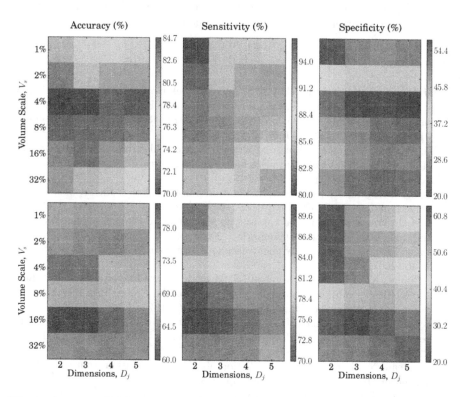

Fig. 3. Accuracy (left), sensitivity (middle) and specificity (right) of the RSCV for CRT response (top) and LBBB (bottom) classification. CRT response prediction has the best accuracy at a spatial scale of 4%, showing high sensitivity at lower scales, and peak specificity at 4%. LBBB identification has peak accuracy, sensitivity and specificity at a scale of 16%, performing best at lower D_j values.

becomes apparent at the larger scales. This distinct pattern is present in most of the patients with LBBB, and contributes to the high sensitivity $(90.2 \pm 12.9\%)$ of LBBB identification, whereas the lower specificity $(63.7 \pm 25.7\%)$ may be due to the presence of more varied deformation patterns amongst patients without LBBB. Similarly, the high CRT response prediction sensitivity $(94.0 \pm 8.1\%)$ suggests responders are generally easily distinguishable by small scale strain patterns, whereas correctly predicting the non-responders remains a challenge given the low specificity $(52.5 \pm 34.2\%)$, and may also be due to the small number of non-responders in the cohort.

With the limited cohort size of 34, we restricted the learning techniques employed to simple methods (PCA and LDA) which would limit over-fitting by minimising the number of parameters. A larger cohort would permit use of more advanced techniques with more parameters, such as manifold learning and non-linear classifiers (e.g. SVMs), as well as reduce the variance in our results. Our framework could also be applied to other cardiac pathologies for which abnormal deformations might be expected, and could be assessed with respect to a healthy subject motion atlas, and in conjunction with clinical indicators to predict disease occurrence or treatment outcome in the future.

References

1. Bai, W., et al.: Beyond the AHA 17-Segment model: motion-driven parcellation of the left ventricle. In: Camara, O., Mansi, T., Pop, M., Rhode, K., Sermesant, M., Young, A. (eds.) STACOM 2015. LNCS, vol. 9534, pp. 13–20. Springer, Heidelberg (2016). doi:10.1007/978-3-319-28712-6_2
2. Bai, W., Shi, W., et al.: A cardiac atlas built from high resolution MR images of 1000 + normal subjects and atlas-based analysis of cardiac shape and motion. Med. Image Anal. **26**(1), 133–145 (2015)
3. Bassingthwaighte, J., van Beek, J.: Lightning and the heart: fractal behavior in cardiac function. Proc. IEEE **76**(6), 693–699 (2002)
4. Bonet, J., Wood, R.: Nonlinear Continuum Mechanics for Finite Element Analysis. Cambridge University Press, Cambridge (2008)
5. Camici, P., Crea, F.: Coronary microvascular dysfunction. N. Engl. J. Med. **356**(8), 830–40 (2007)
6. De Craene, M., Duchateau, N., et al.: SPM to the heart: Mapping of 4D continuous velocities for motion abnormality quantification. In: Proceedings-International Symposium on Biomedical Imaging, pp. 454–457 (2012)
7. Duchateau, N., De Craene, M., et al.: Constrained manifold learning for the characterization of pathological deviations from normality. Med. Image Anal. **16**(8), 1532–1549 (2012)
8. Duchateau, N., Sermesant, M.: Prediction of infarct localization from myocardial deformation. In: STACOM, vol. 9534, pp. 51–59 (2015)
9. Gotte, M., Germans, T., et al.: Myocardial strain and torsion quantified by cardiovascular magnetic resonance tissue tagging: studies in normal and impaired left ventricular function. J. Am. Coll. Cardiol. **48**(10), 2002–2011 (2006)
10. Jackson, T., Sohal, M., et al.: A U-shaped type II contraction pattern in patients with strict left bundle branch block predicts super-response to cardiac resynchronization therapy. Heart Rhythm **11**(10), 1790–1797 (2014)

11. Kirk, J., Kass, D.: Electromechanical dyssynchrony and resynchronization of the failing heart. Circ. Res. **113**(6), 765–776 (2013)
12. Marxen, M., Sled, J., Henkelman, R.: Volume ordering for analysis and modeling of vascular systems. Ann. Biomed. Eng. **37**(3), 542–551 (2009)
13. Peressutti, D., Bai, W., Jackson, T., Sohal, M., Rinaldi, A., Rueckert, D., King, A.: Prospective identification of CRT super responders using a motion atlas and random projection ensemble learning. In: Navab, N., Hornegger, J., Wells, W.M., Frangi, A.F. (eds.) MICCAI 2015. LNCS, vol. 9351, pp. 493–500. Springer, Heidelberg (2015). doi:10.1007/978-3-319-24574-4_59
14. Peressutti, D., Bai, W., Shi, W., Tobon-Gomez, C., Jackson, T., Sohal, M., Rinaldi, A., Rueckert, D., King, A.: Towards left ventricular scar localisation using local motion descriptors. In: Camara, O., Mansi, T., Pop, M., Rhode, K., Sermesant, M., Young, A. (eds.) STACOM 2015. LNCS, vol. 9534, pp. 30–39. Springer, Heidelberg (2016). doi:10.1007/978-3-319-28712-6_4
15. Perperidis, D., Mohiaddin, R., Rueckert, D.: Construction of a 4D statistical atlas of the cardiac anatomy and its use in classification. In: Duncan, J.S., Gerig, G. (eds.) MICCAI 2005. LNCS, vol. 3750, pp. 402–410. Springer, Heidelberg (2005). doi:10.1007/11566489_50
16. Rueckert, D., Sonoda, L., et al.: Nonrigid registration using free-form deformations: application to breast MR images. IEEE Trans. Med. Imaging **18**(8), 712–721 (1999)
17. Sinclair, M., Lee, J., et al.: Microsphere skimming in the porcine coronary arteries: Implications for flow quantification. Microvasc. Res. **100**, 59–70 (2015)
18. Sohal, M., Duckett, S., et al.: A prospective evaluation of cardiovascular magnetic resonance measures of dyssynchrony in the prediction of response to cardiac resynchronization therapy. J. Cardiovasc. Magn. Reson. **16**, 58 (2014)
19. Tian, Y., Zhang, P., et al.: True complete left bundle branch block morphology strongly predicts good response to cardiac resynchronization therapy. Europace **15**(10), 1499–1506 (2013)

3D Reconstruction of Coronary Veins from a Single X-Ray Fluoroscopic Image and Pre-operative MR

Maria Panayiotou[1]([✉]), Daniel Toth[1,3], Tamer Adem[1], Peter Mountney[4], Alexander Brost[5], Jonathan M. Behar[1,2], C. Aldo Rinaldi[2], R. James Housden[1], and Kawal S. Rhode[1]

[1] Division of Imaging Sciences and Biomedical Engineering, King's College London, London, UK
maria.panayiotou@kcl.ac.uk
[2] Deparment of Cardiology, Guy's and St. Thomas' Hospitals NHS Foundation Trust, London, UK
[3] Siemens Healthcare, Ltd, London, UK
[4] Medical Imaging Technologies, Siemens Healthineers, Princeton, NJ, USA
[5] Siemens Healthcare GmbH, Forchheim, Germany

Abstract. Cardiac resynchronization therapy (CRT) is an effective treatment for patients with congestive heart failure and ventricular dyssynchrony. Despite the overall efficacy of CRT, approximately 30% of patients receiving CRT do not improve. One of the main technical problems related to the CRT procedure is inadequate visualisation in X-ray fluoroscopy of the venous anatomy in relation to accurate cardiac chamber visualisation. This paper proposes a novel approach for 3D reconstruction of coronary veins from a single contrast enhanced intraoperative fluoroscopy image. For this application, the method uses backprojection geometry and a Euclidean distance/angle-based cost function. The algorithm is validated on a phantom and five patient datasets, comprising six view-angle orientations for the phantom dataset and two view-angle orientations for each of the patient datasets. Median(interquartile range) 3D-reconstruction accuracies of 1.41(0.55–3.00) mm and 3.28(2.10–4.89) mm were established for the phantom and patient data, respectively. The technique can facilitate careful advancement of the cannulating guide over a guidewire or a diagnostic catheter positioned in the coronary sinus, and consequently, improve the chances of response to CRT.

Keywords: Coronary veins · 3D reconstruction · X-ray fluoroscopy

1 Introduction

Cardiac resynchronization therapy (CRT) has been shown to improve outcomes in a growing subset of patients with congestive heart failure. Although the majority of patients who meet the criteria for CRT under current guidelines derive

T. Mansi et al. (Eds.): STACOM 2016, LNCS 10124, pp. 66–75, 2017.
DOI: 10.1007/978-3-319-52718-5_8

benefit, approximately one-third of patients do not respond to this pacing modality [15]. Most of these failures are due to difficulty accessing the coronary sinus (CS) ostium or advancing the pacing lead into an adequate, stable position [11]. In order to maintain the accuracy of the guidance information, thereby allowing accurate determination of pacing treatment sites, volumetric coronary vein roadmaps overlaid on X-ray fluoroscopy can be used. Coronary vein anatomy can be provided pre-operatively with multislice computed tomography (CT) [9]. However, CT requires an additional use of ionizing radiation and nephrotoxic contrast agents. Cardiac MR (CMR) imaging is also used to depict the anatomy of the venous system of the heart [3], although a high-spatial resolution and longer scan time is required to adequately depict the relatively small coronary vessels.

The standard visualisation method is a 2D X-ray examination using an injection of contrast material, called a venogram. This uses less radiation than CT and is able to visualise vessels that cannot be seen in CMR [5]. Many methods exist for reconstruction of coronary arteries from venograms [4]. The vascular tree can be reconstructed in 3D by triangulation from venograms if at least two views of the coronary vascular tree are obtained. For reconstruction of the vascular tree, however, corresponding vessels must be identified either manually or by use of the vessel hierarchy [6]. Corresponding points along the vessel centerlines can then be established by means of an epipolar-line technique [13]. Paired images for 3D coronary vein reconstruction can be acquired using a biplane X-ray system [2,14], although these are less common than a monoplane system in the clinical setting, and involve increased radiation exposure for both the patient and the clinician. Alternatively, 3D reconstruction of coronary veins can be achieved using a monoplane system. This requires either acquisition of a rotational X-ray sequence [1], which involves a long radiation exposure, or two sequences at arbitrary orientations [10]. Such techniques require both cardiac and respiratory phase matching of the images.

In this paper, a novel semi-automatic approach is presented for 3D reconstruction of coronary veins to overcome the limitations of the already proposed techniques. Unlike all previous techniques the proposed technique can reconstruct the coronary vein centrelines from a single contrast enhanced X-ray fluoroscopic image registered to an MR segmentation. This technique reduces radiation dose and simplifies clinical workflow.

2   Methods

In this section the formation of a 3D model of the coronary veins, reconstructed from a single contrast injected X-ray fluoroscopy image, is described. The workflow of the image analysis framework is illustrated in Fig. 1. Initially, the left ventricle (LV), segmented from preoperative MR, is registered to an intraoperative X-ray fluoroscopic image. The coronary veins are manually annotated on the contrast injected X-ray fluoroscopic image and back-projected to the 3D registered LV mesh. The algorithm makes use of the 3D intersection points between

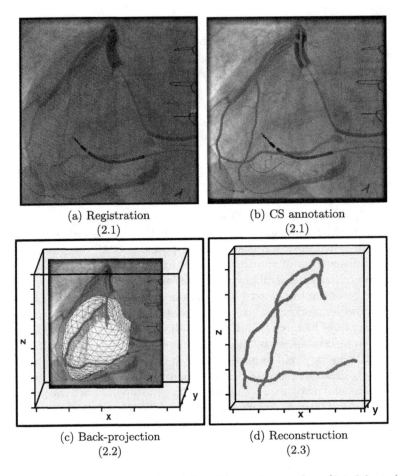

(a) Registration
(2.1)

(b) CS annotation
(2.1)

(c) Back-projection
(2.2)

(d) Reconstruction
(2.3)

Fig. 1. Illustration of the proposed workflow. The section numbers (2.1, 2.2, etc.) refer to the corresponding section numbers in the text.

the back-projected rays and the surface of the LV mesh to search for and locate the position of the coronary veins around the LV surface.

2.1 Registration of LV Mesh and Coronary Vein Annotation

The LV is automatically segmented from pre-procedural MRI. A fully-automatic slice-by-slice segmentation and propagation of the epicardial LV borders in long (two-, three- and four-chamber) and short axis images is computed. The system then generates a mesh of the epicardial cavity that follows the epicardial contours at end diastole, using a model-based segmentation algorithm [8].

A single contrast enhanced (end diastolic, end expiration) frame from the X-ray sequence is automatically selected using Masked-principal component analysis motion gating [12]. As part of the proposed workflow, manual annotation of the centrelines of visible vessels is required on the chosen X-ray image (Fig. 1b). The method requires that the first annotated 2D point should correspond to a point on the posterior side of the LV. This can easily be identified, as the CS ostium is always visible in these images and based on the CS cardiac anatomy it lies on the posterior side of the LV mesh at standard angulations. Finally, a clinical expert manually registers the segmented LV mesh to the X-ray fluoroscopic image using a custom-made visualisation software. This is also done intra-procedurally (Fig. 1a).

2.2 Back-Projection of 2D CS Vessel Annotated Points

X-ray fluoroscopy follows the ideal pinhole camera model that describes the relationship between a 3D point and its corresponding 2D projection onto the image plane. The back-projection of a 2D point in the image plane is a line, called the projection line, calculated using the camera parameters of the X-ray fluoroscopy projective modality [7]. The camera parameters are obtained from the DICOM header of the X-ray images. Using projection geometry, each of the 2D coronary venous positions annotated in Fig. 1b is back-projected to form a 3D line, illustrated in red in Fig. 1c.

2.3 3D Reconstruction of Coronary Veins

To reconstruct the coronary veins in 3D (Fig. 1d), the algorithm uses the 1st reconstructed point and a Euclidean distance/angle-based cost function to determine subsequent points along the vessel. The first 3D point, part of the coronary sinus, lies on the 3D line back-projected from the 1st 2D annotated point. This line intersects the mesh at two points and the correct point must be chosen for the reconstruction. The 1st 3D point is known to be the posterior point. Following the determination of the 1st 3D-reconstructed point, subsequent 3D points are defined according to

$$\mathbf{p}_i = \underset{\mathbf{p}_i}{\operatorname{argmin}}[D(\mathbf{p}_i; \mathbf{p}_{i-1}) + \lambda A(\mathbf{p}_i; \mathbf{p}_{i-1}, \mathbf{p}_{i-2})] \tag{1}$$

where $D(\mathbf{p}_i; \mathbf{p}_{i-1})$ is a function that computes the Euclidean distance between the previously defined 3D point, $\mathbf{p}_{i-1}$, and the candidate points, $\mathbf{p}_i$, as defined in Eq. (2). $A(\mathbf{p}_i; \mathbf{p}_{i-1}, \mathbf{p}_{i-2})$ is a function that computes the angle between $\mathbf{p}_i$ and the two previously defined 3D points, $\mathbf{p}_{i-1}$ and $\mathbf{p}_{i-2}$, as defined by Eq. (3) and illustrated in Fig. 2.

$$D(\mathbf{p}_i; \mathbf{p}_{i-1}) = ||\mathbf{p}_i - \mathbf{p}_{i-1}|| \tag{2}$$

$$A(\mathbf{p}_i; \mathbf{p}_{i-1}, \mathbf{p}_{i-2}) = \begin{cases} 0, & \text{if } i \leq 2 \\ 1 - cos(\theta_i), & \text{otherwise} \end{cases} \tag{3}$$

where $cos(\theta_i) = \frac{\overrightarrow{\mathbf{P}_{i-2}\mathbf{P}_{i-1}} \cdot \overrightarrow{\mathbf{P}_{i-1}\mathbf{P}_i}}{||\overrightarrow{\mathbf{P}_{i-2}\mathbf{P}_{i-1}}||||\overrightarrow{\mathbf{P}_{i-1}\mathbf{P}_i}||}$. λ is the weight given to the distance and angle functions. For this algorithm $\lambda = 2$ was found to favour a smoothly curving path of points, which is important at the edges of the projection where the two distances are very similar.

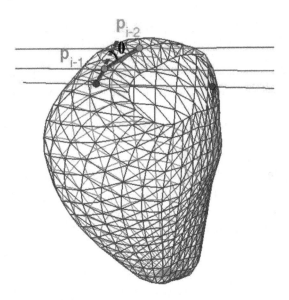

Fig. 2. Illustration of angle, θ, computation. $\mathbf{p}_{i-1}$ and $\mathbf{p}_{i-2}$, illustrated in orange and green colours, respectively, are the two previously defined 3D points. The two blue points are the two candidates for point $\mathbf{p}_i$. (Color figure online)

3   Experiments

3.1   Data Acquisition

The proposed algorithm was quantitatively and qualitatively evaluated on a phantom data set and clinical images acquired from 5 different patients undergoing CRT; these comprised a total of 6 view-angle orientations for the phantom dataset and 2 view-angle orientations for each of the clinical datasets. The phantom experiments were performed to evaluate the proposed approach in a clinical imaging environment with a known ground truth registration. The LV epicardial surface (segmented from an MR image) was 3D printed and wires were attached to model the vascular tree. Intra-operative data were then obtained by acquiring a cone beam CT, which provided the registered LV mesh and 6 X-ray images.

Imaging of three of the clinical datasets was carried out using a monoplane 25 cm flat panel cardiac X-ray system (Philips Allura Xper FD10, Philips Healthcare, Best, The Netherlands) while imaging of the phantom dataset and the remaining two clinical datasets was carried out using a biplane cardiac X-ray system (Artis, syngo X Workplace VC10N, Siemens Healthcare GmbH). This study was approved by our Local Ethics Committee.

3.2   Gold Standard 3D Reconstruction of Coronary Veins

Multiple view-angle orientations were used to obtain a manual ground truth coronary vein reconstruction for each of the tested datasets. Using projection

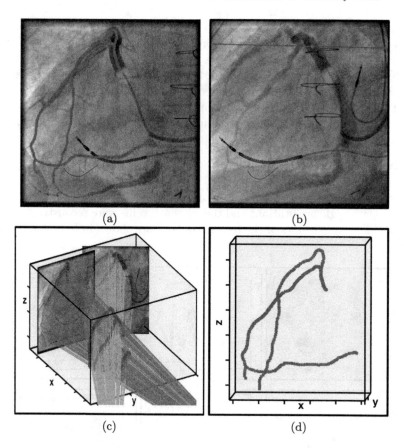

Fig. 3. Illustration of ground truth 3D-reconstruction workflow. (a) 2D manual coronary vein annotation. (b) Use of epipolar line to manually annotate corresponding points in the second view. (c) Back-projection of annotated points from each view angle. (d) 3D coronary vein reconstruction from closest points of intersection between the back-projected rays from each view angle.

geometry, each of the 2D coronary vein positions was carefully annotated (Fig. 3a). Each annotated point was back-projected to form a 3D line, which was then forward projected to generate a 2D epipolar line (Fig. 3b) in a 2nd view that contains the corresponding 2D coronary vein position. For each epipolar line generated, the corresponding coronary vein position was manually detected. Each pair of matching points from the two projection planes was then back-projected (Fig. 3c) to reconstruct the coronary veins in 3D (Fig. 3d).

3.3   Success Rate and Accuracy of Reconstruction

A successfully reconstructed vessel was defined as one that was reconstructed on the correct side of the LV mesh, following a path similar to the gold standard reconstruction. In cases where the wrong path of a vessel was chosen by the algorithm the reconstruction of the specific vessel was considered a failure. Percentage success rates were computed as the proportion of vessels that were successfully reconstructed, for the phantom and patient datasets. The accuracy of the successfully reconstructed vessels, for both the phantom and the patient datasets, was calculated as the mean of the mm distance from each 3D reconstructed point and the nearest point on the gold standard reconstruction.

4   Results

For both the phantom and patient datasets the algorithm was applied on all available view-angle orientations and the coronary veins were reconstructed from each view. Example results of the reconstructions are shown in Figs. 4 and 5. For

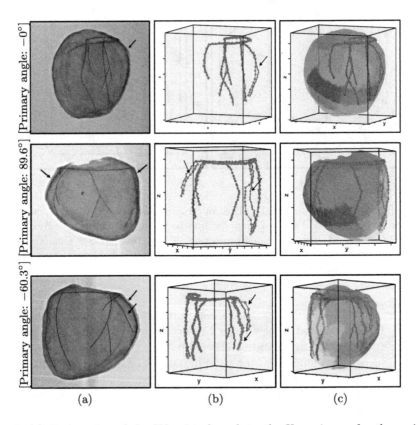

Fig. 4. (a) Registration of the LV printed mesh to the X-ray image for three view-angle orientations. (b) 3D-reconstructed coronary veins (red) and gold standard (blue). The black arrows illustrate the vessels that were unsuccessfully reconstructed by the algorithm. (c) 3D-reconstructed coronary veins overlaid onto the 16 segment colour coded LV epicardium mesh. (Color figure online)

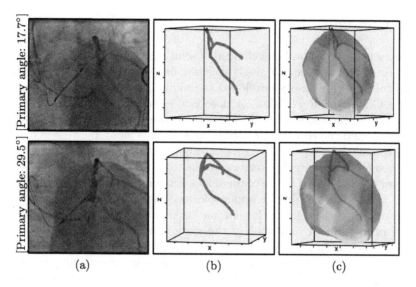

Fig. 5. Example reconstructions of patient data. See the caption to Fig. 4 for the meaning of each image.

the phantom dataset, the gold standard registration of the segmented LV mesh to the X-ray fluoroscopic image is illustrated in Fig. 4a, for the three view angles that included failed reconstructions. Figure 4b illustrates the 3D-reconstructed coronary veins. As part of the planning stage of the CRT procedure the LV surface is divided into 16 segments using the standard 16-segment American Heart Association (AHA) model of the LV for regional analysis. Since clinical decisions for the optimal pacing site are made per segment, Fig. 4c illustrates the 3D-reconstructed coronary veins overlaid on the 16-segment colour coded LV mesh. Figure 5 is a similar illustration, with manual registration of the LV mesh, for one of the patient datasets.

The success rates of the phantom and patient datasets were computed to be 86% and 100%, respectively. The accuracy of the successfully reconstructed vessels is 1.41 mm (inter-quartile range 1.15–2.01 mm) for the phantom and 3.28 mm (2.2–3.72 mm) for patient data. As shown in Fig. 4, the accuracy of the algorithm is reduced for vessels at the edge of the LV projection, and this is where all of the failures occurred. This is because the distance between the two possible reconstructed points is considerably smaller at the edges, and consequently the angle constraint increases in importance resulting in the algorithm failing to choose the correct 3D point. The accuracy of the unsuccessfully reconstructed vessels varies between 3.5–8.19 mm. Even though these vessels are considered failures of the algorithm when compared to the gold standard vessels, they will usually reach the same segments when overlaid onto the 16-segment colour coded mesh given that the average segment width is around 5cm. As a result, this will not negatively affect the guidance during the CRT procedure, as the clinicians only need to know the segments through which the coronary veins pass.

5   Conclusions

This paper presents a novel and clinically useful algorithm for 3D-reconstruction of the coronary veins from a single contrast enhanced intra-procedural X-ray image. Unlike all previously developed techniques, this technique does not disrupt the CRT clinical workflow, it does not require any additional radiation dose to the patient and staff, and there is no requirement to phase match X-ray images or to find the correspondences between points along the vessels in different projections. This technique enables a superior single shot 3D visualisation of the coronary venous system in relation to the regions of the LV. This may enable placement of the LV lead in the optimal location and therefore improve response rates to CRT. It could also be applicable to other procedures, such as percutaneous coronary intervention for chronic total occlusions and radio frequency ablation procedures. A limitation of the method is that the 3D reconstruction may be inaccurate in cases where a vessel is found at the edges of the LV registered mesh. The accuracy is also very dependent on an accurate registration of the mesh to the X-ray. Future work will focus on automating the procedure by replacing the manual centreline annotation step with an automatic coronary vein detection using a deep learning technique, and by using an automatic registration method.

Acknowledgements and Disclaimer. We acknowledge financial support from the Department of Health via the National Institute for Health Research (NIHR) comprehensive Biomedical Research Centre award to Guy's and St Thomas' NHS Foundation Trust in partnership with King's College London, King's College Hospital NHS Foundation Trust and Innovate UK. This work was supported by the Engineering and Physical Sciences Research Council [grant number EP/L505328/1] and Innovate UK. Concepts and information presented are based on research and are not commercially available.

References

1. Blondel, C., Malandain, G., Vaillant, R., Ayache, N.: Reconstruction of coronary arteries from a single rotational x-ray projection sequence. IEEE Trans. Med. Imaging **25**(5), 653–663 (2006)
2. Chen, S.Y.J., Carroll, J., Metz, C., Hoffmann, K.: Method and apparatus for three-dimensional reconstruction of coronary vessels from angiographic images (2000(b))
3. Chiribiri, A., Kelle, S., Götze, S., Kriatselis, C., Thouet, T., Tangcharoen, T., Paetsch, I., Schnackenburg, B., Fleck, E., Nagel, E.: Visualization of the cardiac venous system using cardiac magnetic resonance. American J. Cardiol. **101**(3), 407–412 (2008)
4. Çimen, S., Gooya, A., Grass, M., Frangi, A.: Reconstruction of coronary arteries from x-ray angiography: a review. Med. Image Anal. **32**, 46–68 (2016)
5. Duckett, S., Chiribiri, A., Ginks, M., Sinclair, S., Knowles, B., Botnar, R., Carr White, G., Rinaldi, C., Nagel, E., Razavi, R.: Cardiac MRI to investigate myocardial scar and coronary venous anatomy using a slow infusion of dimeglumine gadobenate in patients undergoing assessment for cardiac resynchronization therapy. J. Magn. Reson. Imaging **33**(1), 87–95 (2011)

6. Guggenheim, N., Doriot, P., Dorsaz, P., Descouts, P., Rutishauser, W.: Spatial reconstruction of coronary arteries from angiographic images. Phys. Med. Biol. **36**(1), 99 (1991)

7. Hartley, R., Zisserman, A.: Multiple View Geometry in Computer Vision, 2nd edn. Cambridge University Press, Cambridge (2004). ISBN: 0521540518

8. Jolly, M.-P., Guetter, C., Lu, X., Xue, H., Guehring, J.: Automatic segmentation of the myocardium in cine MR images using deformable registration. In: Camara, O., Konukoglu, E., Pop, M., Rhode, K., Sermesant, M., Young, A. (eds.) STACOM 2011. LNCS, vol. 7085, pp. 98–108. Springer, Heidelberg (2012). doi:10. 1007/978-3-642-28326-0_10

9. Jongbloed, M.R., Lamb, H.J., Bax, J.J., Schuijf, J.D., de Roos, A., van der Wall, E.E., Schalij, M.J.: Noninvasive visualization of the cardiac venous system using multislice computed tomography. J. Am. Coll. Cardiol. **45**(5), 749–753 (2005)

10. Messenger, J., Chen, S., Carroll, J., Burchenal, J., Kioussopoulos, K., Groves, B.: 3D coronary reconstruction from routine single-plane coronary angiograms: clinical validation and quantitative analysis of the right coronary artery in 100 patients. Int. J. Card. Imaging **16**(6), 413–427 (2000)

11. Moss, A., Hall, W., Cannom, D., Klein, H., Brown, M., Daubert, J., Estes III, N.M., Foster, E., Greenberg, H., Higgins, S.: Cardiac-resynchronization therapy for the prevention of heart-failure events. N. Engl. J. Med. **361**(14), 1329–1338 (2009)

12. Panayiotou, M., King, A., Housden, R., Ma, Y., Cooklin, M., O'Neill, M., Gill, J., Rinaldi, C., Rhode, K.: A statistical method for retrospective cardiac and respiratory motion gating of interventional cardiac x-ray images. Med. phys. **41**(7), 071901 (2014)

13. Parker, D., Pope, D., Van Bree, R., Marshall, H.: Three-dimensional reconstruction of moving arterial beds from digital subtraction angiography. Comput. Biomed. Res. **20**(2), 166–185 (1987)

14. Rivero-Ayerza, M., Jessurun, E., Ramcharitar, S., van Belle, Y., Serruys, P., Jordaens, L.: Magnetically guided left ventricular lead implantation based on a virtual three-dimensional reconstructed image of the coronary sinus. Europace **10**(9), 1042–1047 (2008)

15. Ypenburg, C.E.: Noninvasive imaging in cardiac resynchronization therapy-part 1: selection of patients. Pacing Clin. Electrophysiol. **31**(11), 1475–1499 (2008)

Integrating Atlas and Graph Cut Methods for Left Ventricle Segmentation from Cardiac Cine MRI

Shusil Dangi[1], Nathan Cahill[1,3], and Cristian A. Linte[1,2(✉)]

[1] Chester F. Carlson Center for Imaging Science,
Rochester Institute of Technology, Rochester, NY, USA
{sxd7257,calbme}@rit.edu
[2] Biomedical Engineering, Rochester Institute of Technology, Rochester, NY, USA
[3] Center for Applied and Computational Mathematics,
Rochester Institute of Technology, Rochester, NY, USA

Abstract. Magnetic Resonance Imaging (MRI) has evolved as a clinical standard-of-care imaging modality for cardiac morphology, function assessment, and guidance of cardiac interventions. All these applications rely on accurate extraction of the myocardial tissue and blood pool from the imaging data. Here we propose a framework for left ventricle (LV) segmentation from cardiac cine MRI. First, we segment the LV blood pool using iterative graph cuts, and subsequently use this information to segment the myocardium. We formulate the segmentation procedure as an energy minimization problem in a graph subject to the shape prior obtained by label propagation from an average atlas using affine registration. The proposed framework has been validated on 30 patient cardiac cine MRI datasets available through the STACOM LV segmentation challenge and yielded fast, robust, and accurate segmentation results.

1 Introduction

The World Health Organization (WHO)[1] estimated 17.5 million deaths from cardiovascular diseases in 2012, representing 31% of all mortalities, rendering cardiovascular conditions the main cause of death globally. Hence, the timely diagnosis and treatment follow-up of these pathologies is crucial. High image quality, good tissue contrast, and no ionizing radiation has established MRI as a standard clinical modality for non-invasive assessment of cardiac performance. Cardiac contractile function quantified via the systolic and diastolic volumes, ejection fraction, and myocardial mass represents a reliable diagnostic value and can be computed by segmenting the left (LV) and right (RV) ventricles from cardiac cine MRI. Although manual delineation of the ventricle is deemed as the gold-standard approach, it requires significant time and effort and is highly susceptible to inter- and intra-observer variability. These limitations suggest a need for fast, robust, and accurate semi- or fully-automatic segmentation algorithms.

---

[1] http://www.who.int/mediacentre/factsheets/fs317/en/.

© Springer International Publishing AG 2017
T. Mansi et al. (Eds.): STACOM 2016, LNCS 10124, pp. 76–86, 2017.
DOI: 10.1007/978-3-319-52718-5_9

Various segmentation techniques for cardiac MR images have been proposed in the literature [1]. The image-based approaches with weak or no prior information, such as thresholding, edge-based and region-based approaches, or pixel-based classifications methods, require user interaction for proper segmentation of the ill-defined regions. On the other hand, shape prior deformation models, active shape and appearance models, and atlas-based approaches are more likely to overcome this problem at the expense of manually building a training set.

Multi-atlas based approaches have shown promising results in biomedical image segmentation [2]. However, they rely on a number of computationally demanding and time limiting nonrigid image registration steps followed by label fusion. Hence despite its accuracy, it has experienced minimal to no adoption in actual clinical applications primarily due to its complexity, high dependence on parameters variability, and computational demands.

On the other hand, combinatorial optimization based graph-cut techniques are fast and guaranteed to produce results within a known factor of the global minimum, for some special classes of functions (termed as regular functions) [3] and have proved to be powerful tools for image segmentation. Moreover, adding a shape constraint into the graph cut framework has been shown to improve the cardiac image segmentation results significantly [4–6]. However, these methods require a manual input to introduce a shape constraint at the right location in the image.

In this work, we leverage the performance of the graph cut framework and augment it by incorporating shape constraints in the form of an average atlas-based segmentation of the anatomy whose label was generated and propagated using a single affine registration. Subsequently, we iteratively refine the segmentation using techniques similar to those described in [7,8], to obtain an accurate and robust segmentation of the myocardium. Hence, we do not require any manual input to introduce shape constraint into the graph-cut framework and simultaneously take advantage of the prior knowledge in the form of atlas-based segmentation requiring affine as opposed to nonrigid registration, which is more computationally efficient and less sensitive to parameters variability.

2   Methodology

Whole heart cine MRI images are generated by stacking 2D+T short-axis slices acquired during a single breath hold. Since this acquisition approach introduces an intensity difference between the slices, as well as slice misalignments, we can follow one of two approaches to segment tha data: one approach is to implement a slice motion correction protocol to realign the slices into a coherent 3D volume. The other approach, also implemented here, resorts to slice-wise processing and segmentation instead of a 3D segmentation.

Another challenge is the ill-defined contrast of the LV myocardium in MR images, which makes the image-driven segmentation difficult. As such, to obtain better segmentation of the apical and basal regions, we exploit the prior knowledge in the form of an average atlas. The proposed methodology formulates the segmentation problem in the context of a graph based energy minimization framework. The blood pool is first segmented using an iterative graph cut technique; then, this information is used to segment the myocardium.

2.1 Data Preprocessing

This study is conducted on 30 cardiac cine-MR images taken from the DETER-MINE [9] cohort available as a part of the STACOM Cardiac Atlas Segmentation Challenge Project database[2]. The semi-automatically segmented images obtained by applying the method described in [10] accompany the dataset and serves as gold-standard for assessing the proposed segmentation technique.

We select a reference patient volume with good contrast, average size, and preferred LV-RV orientation. All patient volumes are rotated about the z-axis (i.e., slice-encoding direction) to roughly align their orientation with that of the reference patient using the DICOM Image Orientation Patient (IPP) field. The region of interest (ROI) (in the xy-plane) enclosing the left and right ventricles is extracted using the method described in [11] by correlating the 2D motion images generated from the 3D volumes across the cardiac cycle. The only manual input required by our algorithm is the start and end slices of the LV, such that the ROI is restricted in the z-direction, preventing over/under segmentation of slices that do not belong to the desired anatomy. The patient volumes are cropped to the above ROI, and, to compensate for any intensity differences (due to the slice-wise acquisition), each slice is normalized (0–255) prior to further processing.

2.2 Atlas Generation

The cropped 3D volumes (at the end diastole phase) for all patients are first histogram matched and then affinely registered to the reference patient image volume using the intensity based Nelder-Meade downhill simplex algorithm [12] available in SimpleITK. The resulting 3D affine transforms are applied to the respective ground truth segmentations. The transformed volumes and transformed ground truths are then averaged to obtain an average appearance atlas and a probabilistic atlas, respectively (Fig. 1).

The average appearance atlas is registered to a test volume using intensity-based affine registration. The resulting registration transformation is used to transform the myocardial probabilistic label to the test data, which, in turn, serves as a shape constraint for the graph cut framework.

2.3 LV Blood Pool Segmentation Using Iterative Graph Cuts

To leverage the 3D LV geometry, we use the blood pool (BP) segmentation of a given slice to help refine the BP ROI in the neighboring slices. As such, we first segment the BP from the mid-slice, followed by its neighboring slices, and proceed accordingly, until the complete volume is segmented.

---

[2] http://www.cardiacatlas.org.

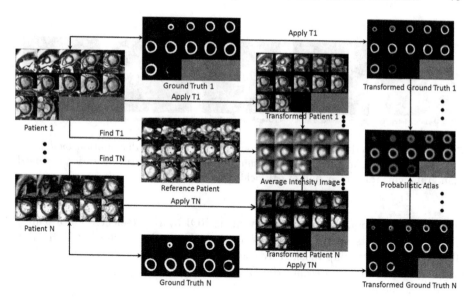

Fig. 1. All patient images are affinely registered to the reference patient, and the obtained optimum transformation is applied to the corresponding ground truth images. An average intensity image is obtained by averaging the intensities of all transformed patient images, while, the averaging of the transformed ground truth images yields a probabilistic atlas.

Intensity Distribution Model. The myocardium probability map for each slice is normalized and inverted to produce the probability map corresponding to the blood pool (BP) and background (BG). The resulting BP/BG probability map is thresholded at 0.5 and the inner connected component is isolated to obtain the high confidence BP ROI. Otsu thresholding [13] is applied within this ROI to obtain the initial BP region. The intensity values within this extracted BP region are then fitted to a Gaussian distribution to generate the BP intensity model.

A binary mask enclosing the myocardium is obtained by thresholding the myocardial probability map at a very small value (i.e. 0.1). Holes in the binary mask are filled to obtain a ROI enclosing the BP, myocardium, and BG. To generate the BG intensity model, we fit the intensity values within the ROI, excluding the initial BP region, to a Gaussian Mixture Model (GMM) comprising two Gaussians. Figure 2a shows the resulting BP log-likelihood map.

Note that we propose the Gaussian distribution for modeling intensity noise in MR images instead of a more appropriate Rician distribution [14]; this simplifies our model and is a good approximation when the signal-to-noise ratio is high.

Blood Pool/Background Probabilistic Map. To obtain a ROI that includes the myocardium and BP, we threshold the myocardial probability map at 0.5,

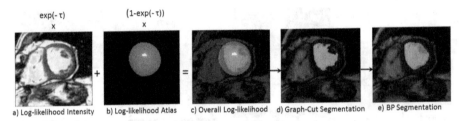

a) Log-likelihood Intensity   b) Log-likelihood Atlas   c) Overall Log-likelihood   d) Graph-Cut Segmentation   e) BP Segmentation

Fig. 2. Log-likelihood image obtained from: (a) the intensity distribution model, (b) the BP probabilistic map, (c) weighted sum of (a) and (b); (d) segmentation obtained from graph cut, (e) convex hull of (d) yields the BP segmentation.

fill in the blood pool, and erode the resulting ROI by 15% (selected empirically) of the radius of its smallest circumscribed circle to obtain the BP ROI. The BP/BG probability map masked by the BP-ROI represents the BP probability map, and its inverse represents the BG probability map. Figure 2b shows the BP log-likelihood map.

Graph-Cut Segmentation. We construct a graph with each node (i.e., pixel) connected to its east, west, north, and south neighbors. Two special terminal nodes representing two classes — the source (blood pool), and the sink (background) — are added to the graph and all other nodes are connected to each terminal node. The segmentation is formulated as an energy minimization problem over the space of optimal labelings f:

$$E(f) = \sum_{p \in \mathcal{P}} D_p(f_p) + \sum_{\{p,q\} \in \mathcal{N}} V_{p,q}(f_p, f_q), \tag{1}$$

where the first term represents the data energy that reduces the disagreement between the labeling f_p given the observed data at every pixel $p \in P$, and the second term represents the smoothness energy that forces pixels p and q defined by a set of interacting pair $\mathcal{N}$ (in our case, the neighboring pixels) towards the same label.

The data energy term is represented by the terminal link (t-link) between each node and the source (or sink), which is defined as the weighted sum of the log probabilities of the intensity distribution model and the probabilistic map corresponding to the BP (or BG):

$$D_p(f_p) = exp\,(\tau) * [-lnPr(I_p|f_p)] + (1 - exp\,(-\tau)) * [-lnPr(f_p)] \tag{2}$$

where, τ is the iteration number, $Pr(I_p|f_p)$ is the likelihood of observing the intensity I_p given that pixel p belongs to class f_p, and $Pr(f_p)$ is the prior probability for class f_p obtained from the BP/BG probability map. The log-likelihood difference between BP and BG labels for $\tau = 1$ is shown in Fig. 2c. The intensity likelihood term (first term) allows the expansion of the BP region in the first few iterations, whereas the prior probability map (second term) restricts its "spilling" (due to over-segmentation) in subsequent iterations.

The smoothness energy term is computed over the links between neighboring nodes (n-links), which are weighted based on their intensity similarity:

$$V_{p,q}(f_p, f_q) = \begin{cases} \tau * exp\left(-\frac{|I_p - I_q|}{\tau}\right) & \text{if } f_p = f_q \\ 0 & \text{if } f_p \neq f_q \end{cases} \qquad (3)$$

where I is the pixel intensity. To avoid the "spilling" of the BP into the myocardium or BG, the smoothness term changes with each iteration, such that, in order for the neighboring pixels to be assigned to the same label during the current iteration, their intensities must be closer than in the previous iteration.

Once weights are assigned to all edges in the graph, the minimum cut equivalent to the maximum flow is identified via the α-expansion algorithm described in [15]. This approach yields the labeling (graph-cut) that minimizes the global energy of the graph that corresponds to the optimal segmentation (Fig. 2d). Lastly, the convex hull applied to the graph-cut result constitutes the final BP segmentation, such that, the papillary muscles are included within the BP (Fig. 2e).

Myocardial Probability Map Refinement. The myocardial probability map is thresholded at 0.5, and the inner hollow circular region representing the BP is extracted. The signed distance map corresponding to the boundary of the extracted BP region is affinely registered to the signed distance map generated from the boundary of the graph-cut extracted BP (Sect. 2.3) segmentation. The optimum affine transformation that minimizes the sum of squared differences between the two distance maps is applied to the myocardial probability map, such that, it fits the shape of the segmented BP.

Iterative Refinement. The latest BP segmentation obtained from the graph cut is used to update the intensity distribution model. The refined myocardial probability map is used to construct a new BP/BG probability map. The pixels within the latest BP segmentation are assigned very high likelihood (for belonging to the BP), and hence their labels do not change. An updated BP segmentation is obtained via another graph cut operating on the new graph energy configuration. This iterative process is repeated until the changes in the affine transform parameters for the myocardium probability map are below a predefined threshold; this iterative process usually converges within three iterations. Upon convergence, the convex hull defined by the latest segmentation result constitutes the final BP segmentation. Figure 3 illustrates the iterative refinement process.

2.4   Myocardium Segmentation

The information from the BP segmentation along with the refined myocardial probability map is used to segment the myocardium.

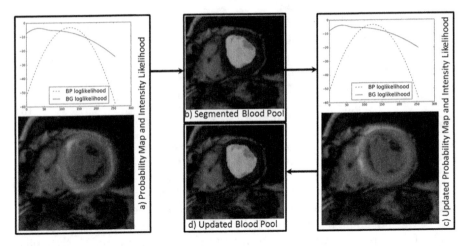

Fig. 3. (a) Probability map and intensity distribution model for current iteration, (b) BP segmentation obtained from graph cut using (a), (c) updated probability map and intensity distribution model obtained using (b), (d) new BP segmentation obtained from graph cut using (c).

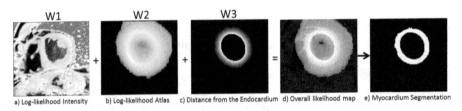

Fig. 4. Log-likelihood image obtained from: (a) the intensity distribution model, (b) the refined myocardium probability map, (c) distance from the endocardium; (d) the weighted sum (w1, w2, and w3) of (a), (b), and (c), respectively; (e) final myocardium segmentation obtained from graph cuts

Intensity Distribution Model. We select a ROI in each slice based on the refined probability map, and we match the histogram of the pixel intensities within this ROI to the histogram of the mid-slice. We select the mid-slices (i.e. no apical/basal slices) to obtain a single intensity distribution model for the whole volume. The intensities of the pixels within the refined myocardial mask with probability higher than 0.5 are fitted to a single Gaussian GMM to obtain the myocardium intensity distribution model. Similarly, the intensities of the remaining pixels are fitted to a three Gaussian GMM to obtain the BG intensity distribution model. Figure 4a shows the log-likelihood map for the myocardium.

Distance from the Endocardial Border. The endocardial border is obtained from the outer edge of the final BP segmentation (Fig. 2e). The knowledge that myocardium should be closer to the endocardial border is encoded in the data term represented by the truncated distance map (empirically selected as 10 pixels). This constraint increases the likelihood of pixels near the endocardial border to be labeled as myocardium, while reducing this likelihood for the pixels located further away. Furthermore, to prevent the BP region from being labeled as myocardium, it is assigned the lowest likelihood value (Fig. 4c).

Graph-Cut Segmentation. A graph is constructed similar to the formulation described in Sect. 2.3, but this time to classify the myocardial rather than blood pool pixels. The data term is defined as the weighted sum of the intensity distribution model, refined myocardial probability map (as described in Sect. 2.3 and Fig. 4b), and the distance from endocardial border, with increasing relative influence, respectively. The smoothness term varies spatially according to the intensity difference between the neighboring pixes, as discussed in Sect. 2.3. The minimum cut in the graph yields the final myocardium segmentation (Fig. 4e).

3 Results

The proposed algorithm was implemented in Python and required 45 seconds on average to segment the BP and myocardium from cine MRI volumes on an Intel® Xenon® 3.60 GHz 32GB RAM PC.

Adhering to the collated results reported for the LV segmentation challenge in [16], we evaluated our segmentation on 30 patient datasets according to the following metrics: dice index, jaccard index, sensitivity, specificity, positive predictive value (PPV), and negative predictive value (NPV) [16]. To maintain approximately equal number of myocardium and non-myocardium pixels for evaluation, such that the NPV conveys some useful information, we dilated each slice of the myocardium region, for the provided gold standard segmentation, by one fourth of the radius of the disk with equivalent area. The segmentation results for a patient dataset are overlaid onto each slice of the patient volume and shown in Fig. 5a. Figure 5b shows a visual comparison of our segmentation results vis-à-vis the provided semi-automated segmentation serving as a gold-standard. The metrics are summarized in Table 1 for all slices together, as well as for the mid-slices and apical/basal slices (first and last two slices, respectively) separately.

4 Discussion, Conclusion, and Future Work

Our validation experiments show that the overall segmentation results are comparable to those reported in [17]. Specifically, the mean values for reported indices were: dice index — 0.68 to 0.88, jaccard index — 0.53 to 0.80, sensitivity — 0.63 to 0.90, specificity — 0.73 to 0.99, PPV — 0.66 to 0.96, and NPV — 0.81 to 0.94. However, it should be noted that the metrics reported in [17] were evaluated against the consensus segmentation estimated based on the participating seven raters (manual and automatic) obtained using STAPLE algorithm on

Table 1. Evaluation of our segmentation results against the provided gold-standard semi-automated segmentation for the mid-slices, apical/basal slices according to Dice Index, Jaccard Index, Sensitivity, Specificity, PPV, and NPV.

Assessment metric	Mid-slices	Apical/Basal-slices	All slices
Dice Index	0.811 ± 0.068	0.568 ± 0.241	0.740 ± 0.180
Jaccard Index	0.687 ± 0.091	0.433 ± 0.222	0.613 ± 0.183
Sensitivity	0.854 ± 0.104	0.596 ± 0.268	0.783 ± 0.195
Specificity	0.788 ± 0.103	0.725 ± 0.180	0.770 ± 0.134
PPV	0.789 ± 0.079	0.714 ± 0.160	0.767 ± 0.114
NPV	0.866 ± 0.086	0.640 ± 0.224	0.800 ± 0.174

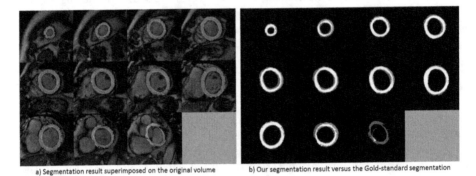

a) Segmentation result superimposed on the original volume   b) Our segmentation result versus the Gold-standard segmentation

Fig. 5. (a) Final myocardium segmentation of all slices of a patient dataset (shown in blue) superimposed with the patient volume (shown in red); (b) Final myocardium segmentation assessed against the provided gold-standard semi-automatic segmentation; white regions represent true positives, red regions represent false negatives, and blue regions represent false positives. (Color figure online)

18 test patient datasets, whereas ours is compared against the provided semi-automatic gold standard segmentation on 30 training patient datasets. Hence, the metrics provide only an approximate estimate of our algorithm's performance compared to the ones that participated in the challenge. Moreover, the average segmentation time of 45 s per volume for an unoptimized code in Python presents a great potential of our algorithm for near real-time clinical applications.

Since the BP region in the mid-slices are better defined than in the apical/basal slices, the segmentation results are consistently better for the mid-slices. We also observed that the slice-wise processing and iterative refinement might compromise the segmentation of the apical/basal slices due to ill-defined BP regions, suggesting the need for special processing for these slices.

As part of our future work, we plan to automate the ROI detection in z-direction to eliminate the manual input required by our algorithm. In addition, instead of using a constant truncating endocardial distance constraint, we plan to use image-derived edge information to enable spatially varying truncating distances to improve the myocardium segmentation. Similarly, we will study the effect of selecting different thresholds for the probability maps, weight variability on the likelihood terms and, in turn, on the final myocardium segmentation. Lastly, we plan to extend the work and evaluate the segmentation performance on all 100 patient datasets and report performance according to the metrics outlined above.

References

1. Petitjean, C., Dacher, J.N.: A review of segmentation methods in short axis cardiac MR images. Med. Image Anal. **15**(2), 169–184 (2011)
2. Iglesias, J.E., Sabuncu, M.R.: Multi-atlas segmentation of biomedical images: a survey. Med. Image Anal. **24**(1), 205–219 (2015)
3. Kolmogorov, V., Zabin, R.: What energy functions can be minimized via graph cuts? IEEE Trans. Pattern Anal. Mach. Intell. **26**(2), 147–159 (2004)
4. Grosgeorge, D., Petitjean, C., Dacher, J.N., Ruan, S.: Graph cut segmentation with a statistical shape model in cardiac MRI. Comput. Vis. Image Underst. **117**(9), 1027–1035 (2013)
5. Freedman, D., Zhang, T.: Interactive graph cut based segmentation with shape priors. In: Proceedings - 2005 IEEE Computer Society Conference on Computer Vision and Pattern Recognition, CVPR 2005, vol. 1, pp. 755–762 (2005)
6. Mahapatra, D.: Cardiac image segmentation from cine cardiac MRI using graph cuts and shape priors. J. Digit. Imaging **26**(4), 721–730 (2013)
7. Slabaugh, G., Unal, G.: Graph cuts segmentation using an elliptical shape prior. In: Proceedings - International Conference on Image Processing, ICIP, vol. 2, pp. 1222–1225 (2005)
8. Vu, N., Manjunath, B.S.: Shape prior segmentation of multiple objects with graph cuts. In: 26th IEEE Conference on Computer Vision and Pattern Recognition, CVPR (2008)
9. Kadish, A.H., Bello, D., Finn, J.P., Bonow, R.O., Schaechter, A., Subacius, H., Albert, C., Daubert, J.P., Fonseca, C.G., Goldberger, J.J.: Rationale and design for the defibrillators to reduce risk by magnetic resonance imaging evaluation (determine) trial. J. Cardiovasc. Electrophysiol. **20**(9), 982–987 (2009)
10. Li, B., Liu, Y., Occleshaw, C.J., Cowan, B.R., Young, A.A.: In-line automated tracking for ventricular function with magnetic resonance imaging. JACC: Cardiovasc. Imaging **3**(8), 860–866 (2010)
11. Ben-Zikri, Y.K., Linte, C.A.: A robust automated left ventricle region of interest localization technique using a cardiac cine MRI atlas (2016)
12. Nelder, J.A., Mead, R.: A simplex method for function minimization. Comput. J. **7**(4), 308–313 (1965)
13. Otsu, N.: A threshold selection method from gray-level histograms. IEEE Transactions on Systems, Man, and Cybernetics **9**(1), 62–66 (1979)
14. Gudbjartsson, H., Patz, S.: The rician distribution of noisy MRI data. Magn. Reson. Med. **34**(6), 910–914 (1995)
15. Boykov, Y., Veksler, O., Zabih, R.: Fast approximate energy minimization via graph cuts. IEEE Trans. PAMI **23**, 1222–1239 (2001)

16. Suinesiaputra, A., Cowan, B.R., Al-Agamy, A.O., Elattar, M.A., Ayache, N., Fahmy, A.S., Khalifa, A.M., Medrano-Gracia, P., Jolly, M.P., Kadish, A.H., Lee, D.C., Margeta, J., Warfield, S.K., Young, A.A.: A collaborative resource to build consensus for automated left ventricular segmentation of cardiac MR images. Med. Image Anal. **18**(1), 50–62 (2014)
17. Suinesiaputra, A., et al.: Left ventricular segmentation challenge from cardiac MRI: a collation study. In: Camara, O., Konukoglu, E., Pop, M., Rhode, K., Sermesant, M., Young, A. (eds.) STACOM 2011. LNCS, vol. 7085, pp. 88–97. Springer, Heidelberg (2012). doi:10.1007/978-3-642-28326-0_9

Cartan Frame Analysis of Hearts with Infarcts

Damien Goblot[1], Mihaela Pop[2], and Kaleem Siddiqi[1(✉)]

[1] School of Computer Science and Centre for Intelligent Machines,
McGill University, Quebec, Canada
`siddiqi@cim.mcgill.ca`
[2] Department of Medical Biophysics, Sunnybrook Research Institute,
University of Toronto, Toronto, Canada

Abstract. Muscle fibers in healthy hearts follow a regular geometry, with streamlines that lie along close to parallel helical curves. This regularity is disrupted in the presence of myocardial infarction which results in a loss of contractile function due to the necrosis of myocytes and the build up of collagen. However, intermediate situations also exist with partly functional surrounding border zones. The precise manner in which fiber geometry is remodeled following the occurrence of an infarct is not known. Here we demonstrate the promise of Cartan frame fitting to diffusion magnetic resonance images of the heart to address this question. We use the error of fit of these models to the first principal eigen vector of the diffusion tensor to capture the degree of local fiber coherence. The first study of its kind in application to myocardial infarction, our experiments on porcine hearts reveal measures to assess damage that are complementary to existing scalar ones, such as the apparent diffusion coefficient or the fractional anisotropy. Cartan frame fitting provides valuable additional information about local fiber geometry.

1 Introduction

In North America alone there are almost half a million sudden deaths each year due to heart defects [16]. In patients suffering from structural heart disease over 85% of the cases arise from myocardial infarction (MI). Following MI, the deposition of collagen (the main component of cardiac connective tissue) in the scar triggers a prolonged ventricular remodelling process [11]. Studies have shown that by 4 weeks after the occurrence of an infarct, mature fibrosis has replaced necrotic myocytes [3,5]. This deposition of collagen is heterogeneous due to surviving blood vessels which continue to supply oxygen to the peri-infarct area [2], resulting in a mixture of viable and necrotic cells to form a border zone (BZ), which in turn can generate lethal arrhythmias [12]. Developing non-invasive methods to characterize the BZ has been the focus of many research groups.

A common strategy is to use diffusion-weighted (DW) imaging to provide scalar parametric maps of the apparent diffusion coefficient (ADC) and the fractional anisotropy (FA), which can identify in vivo scar areas in patients with

© Springer International Publishing AG 2017
T. Mansi et al. (Eds.): STACOM 2016, LNCS 10124, pp. 87–95, 2017.
DOI: 10.1007/978-3-319-52718-5_10

prior-infarction [15] and structural changes in infarcted porcine hearts, ex vivo [8,14]. The molecular diffusion of water molecules reflects microstructural tissue integrity and there is a gradual loss of fiber coherence in the ischemic BZ and dense scar regions due to collagen deposition. The loss in fiber coherence leads to a decrease in FA in these regions, while the deposition of collagen combined with increased extracellular spacing results in elevated ADC values. This relationship between ADC and FA is illustrated by the examples in Fig. 1, with the ADC map (top left) showing increased diffusion (yellowish tones) in the scar tissue, and the FA map showing a corresponding decrease (dark blue tones) in anisotropy (top middle) in an infarcted pig heart.

In healthy mammalian hearts myofibers are known to lie along helical curves, an arrangement that is critical for normal mechanical and electrophysiological function [4]. Numerous mathematical models for this arrangement have been proposed in the literature including [1,6,9,10]. Much less is known, however, about the manner in which heart wall myofibers rearrange in the presence of infarcts. Qualitatively, in healthy regions the fibers maintain a smoothly varying helical pattern, as revealed by tractography (Fig. 1, bottom left), while at locations affected by the infarct their geometry is much more chaotic (Fig. 1, bottom right).

Motivated by the above considerations, we propose to use the error of fit of Cartan frames to fiber orientation data from DW images as a measure of fiber orientation incoherence. We demonstrate the association of regions with a high error of fit with an infarct, while simultaneously providing parametric maps of fiber geometry in healthy tissue. We provide experimental results on several porcine hearts with infarcts and one that is healthy. As a preview of these results, Fig. 1 (top right) shows that regions of low error of fit (dark blue) are consistent with the healthy tissue, as corroborated by the ADC and FA maps. Regions with high error of fit (yellow tones) correspond well with the infarcted regions, where fiber incoherence is expected, but additionally include locations near the epithelial and endothelial linings.

2   Methods

2.1   Modeling Fiber Geometry via Connection Forms

We utilize the methods of [7] to describe the geometry of fiber orientation in the heart wall via rotations of a frame field that is fit to the DW data. Let a point $x = \sum_i x_i e_i \in \mathbf{R}^3$ be expressed in terms of e_1, e_2, e_3, the natural basis for $\mathbf{R}^3$. We define a right-handed orthonormal frame field $f_1, f_2, f_3 : \mathbf{R}^3 \to \mathbf{R}^3$. Each frame axis can be expressed by the rigid rotation $f_i = \sum_j a_{ij} e_j$, where $A = \{a_{ij}\} \in \mathbf{R}^{3 \times 3}$ is a differentiable attitude matrix such that $A^{-1} = A^T$. Treating f_i and e_j as symbols, we can write

$$\begin{bmatrix} f_1 \ f_2 \ f_3 \end{bmatrix}^T = A \begin{bmatrix} e_1 \ e_2 \ e_3 \end{bmatrix}^T. \tag{1}$$

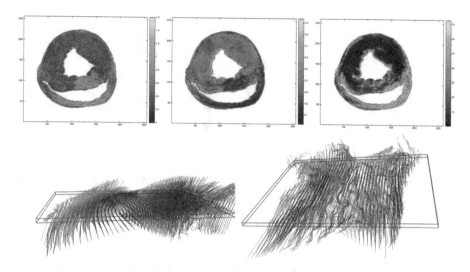

Fig. 1. Ex vivo diffusion imaging of a pig heart. Top: The ADC map (left), with regions of high diffusion shown in shades of yellow, the FA map (middle), with regions of low FA shown in darker blue and the error of fit in degrees generated by fitting 1-forms (right). Bottom: Streamline tractography seeded in a healthy region of the LV wall (left) and in a region of the septum affected by the infarct (right). Both tractography results are visualized from a circumferential direction. See text for a discussion. (Color figure online)

Since each e_i is constant, the differential geometry of the frame field is completely characterized by A. Taking the exterior derivative on both sides, we have

$$\mathrm{d}\left[f_1\ f_2\ f_3\right]^T = (\mathrm{d}A)\, A^{-1}\left[f_1\ f_2\ f_3\right]^T = C\left[f_1\ f_2\ f_3\right]^T, \qquad (2)$$

where d denotes the exterior derivative, and $C = (\mathrm{d}A)\,A^{-1} = \{c_{ij}\} \in \mathbf{R}^{3\times3}$ is the Maurer-Cartan matrix of connection forms c_{ij}. Writing f_i as symbols, (2) is to be understood as $\mathrm{d}f_i = \sum_j c_{ij} f_j$. The Maurer-Cartan matrix is skew symmetric with zeros as diagonal entries so there are at most 3 independent, non-zero 1-forms: c_{12}, c_{13}, and c_{23}. 1-forms operate on vectors through *contraction*, written as $\mathrm{d}w\langle v\rangle \in \mathbf{R}$ for a general 1-form $\mathrm{d}w = \sum_i w_i \mathrm{d}e_i$ and vector v on $\mathbf{R}^3$, which yields $\mathrm{d}w\langle v\rangle = \sum_i w_i \mathrm{d}e_i\langle\sum_j v_j e_j\rangle = \sum_i w_i v_i$, since $\mathrm{d}e_i\langle e_j\rangle = \delta_{ij}$, where δ_{ij} is the Kronecker delta. It turns out that the space of linear models for smoothly varying frame fields is parametrized by the 1-forms c_{ij}. Since only 3 unique non-zero combinations of c_{ij} are possible, there are in total 9 connection parameters c_{ijk}. These coefficients express the rate of turn of the frame vector f_i towards f_j when x moves in the direction f_k. With f_1 taken as the local orientation of a fiber and f_3 taken to be the component of the heart wall normal orthogonal to f_1, Fig. 2 illustrates the connection parameter c_{123} describing the rotation of fibers in the direction of a transmural penetration of the heart wall.

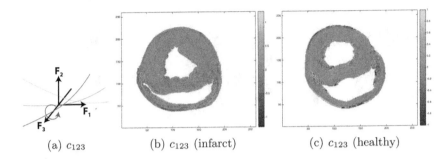

(a) c_{123} (b) c_{123} (infarct)   (c) c_{123} (healthy)

Fig. 2. Connection forms measure the local rotations of the frame axes f_1, f_2, f_3. Here we focus on the contraction of the 1-form c_{12} on the frame axis f_3 and compare its values in a short axis slice of a pig heart with an infarct (middle) with those in a short axis slice from a healthy pig heart (right). See text for a discussion.

Cartan frame fitting applies to smoothly rotating frame fields. In the presence of infarcts fiber orientation coherence is lost and the fitting errors using this method increase (Fig. 1 middle left). We shall exploit this association of frame field fitting error with fiber incoherence.

2.2   Cartan Frame Fitting and Error Analysis

At each voxel we use the first principal eigen vector of a diffusion tensor reconstruction to represent the fiber orientation as f_1. We then estimate the heart wall normal as the gradient of the distance function to the boundary of the myocardium and take its component orthogonal to f_1 to be f_3. f_2 is then taken to be their cross product. To find the 9 connection parameters at each voxel we use Nelder-Mead optimization to minimize a fitting energy. This energy is defined at each voxel as the average of the angle between the measured orientation from DW data at each voxel in a local neighborhood and that given by rotating the frame field by a particular set of connections. Once this method has converged to a set of connection parameters the fitting error at the voxel is taken to be this average angular error between the model and the data.

2.3   Pig Hearts

In this study we used healthy and infarcted porcine hearts. The hearts were freshly excised, suspended in a plexiglass phantom filled with fluorinert to eliminate artifacts and placed in an MR head coil for ex vivo imaging. All DW-MR studies were performed on a dedicated 1.5T GE Signa Excite scanner using a custom FSE pulse sequence. We used the following MR parameters: $TE = 35$ ms, $TR = 700$ ms, echo train length $= 2$, b value $= 0$ for the un-weighted MR images and b value $= 500$ s/mm^2 when the 7 diffusion gradients were applied, respectively. We used a 256×256 k-space, FOV $= 10$–16 cm and a slice thickness of 1.2 mm, yielding a sub-millimetric voxel size. From each heart, select samples containing an infarct were cut to align with the short-axis view of the MR images and prepared for histopathology to confirm the collagen deposition in the infarct area. The details of the methods used to generate the chronic infarcts are presented in [8].

3   Results and Discussion

Reconstruction and Filtering. We used an established Rician smoothing method to reduce noise in the diffusion images [13]. The parameters for this non-local filtering method guided by voxel to voxel similarity were tuned to prevent over-smoothing. We used the publicly available MedInria software to carry out the filtering, and to then reconstruct the diffusion tensor from the raw diffusion weighted scans, from which fiber orientations were extracted as the first principal eigen vector. We used a threshold on the FA map as a mask to restrict further processing.

Comparison with Histology. We first applied a combination of linear and non-linear registration transformations using functions readily available in Matlab, in particular *imregtform*, to align histological slices to their corresponding DW slices. We then compared ADC maps with Cartan frame fitting-based error of fit maps. Supplementing the earlier results in Fig. 1, Fig. 3 shows the ADC map (left) the error of fit map in degrees (middle) and a histology image (right) for a different slice of the dataset in Fig. 1 (top row) and for a selected region from a different infarcted pig heart (middle row). The histology images show intact myocytes in the normal tissue and altered tissue microstructure in the infarcted zones. As depicted by the Masson Trichrome stain, the ischemic border zones (BZ) had collagen fibrils interdigitated between viable myocytes. In the dense scar areas, necrotic myocytes were completely replaced by mature fibrosis (the final product of collagen degradation), resulting in a loss of myocardial anisotropy. The bottom row shows tractography results for these cases. As before there is qualitatively good agreement between regions with high ADC values and regions with high error of fit (yellowish tones). The results also show regions of viable tissue (greenish tones in the error of fit maps) within the infarcted areas, which is corroborated by the tractography results. In particular, there appear to be regions of coherent fibers within the septum of the first heart (third row left) and the LV wall of the second heart (third row right and bottom row left).

Quantitative Results. Given the association between ADC and our error of frame fit, it is natural to compare these measures quantitatively throughout the myocardium. We did so for the 5 infarcted porcine hearts we analyzed by computing Dice coefficients to describe the overlap, in the following manner. For the same heart let A be the set of voxels with ADC value >0.6 and let B be the set of voxels with error of fit $>15°$. The ADC threshold is chosen based on results in [8] which demonstrate the mean ADC value of normal tissue for these DW scans to be below 0.5 with the mean value of border zone or scar tissue regions being above 0.6. The error of fit threshold was chosen by empirical

92   D. Goblot et al.

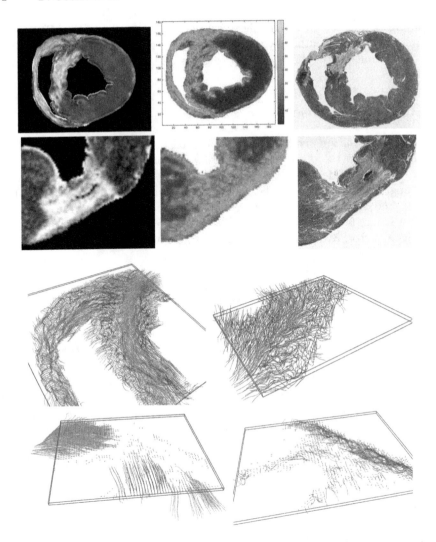

Fig. 3. We now register the histology to the DW images and show the ADC map (left) the error of fit (middle) and the registered histological image (right) for a different slice of the dataset in Fig. 1 (top row) and for a zoomed-in region of a different pig heart with an infarct (second row). The corresponding tractography results are shown in the third row. The bottom row shows tractography for the second case while seeding separately from locations with low error of fit (left) and high error of fit (right). (Color figure online)

considerations, but modest changes to it did not significantly alter the standard Dice coefficient, computed as $A \cap B / A \cup B$, or a modified coefficient computed as $A \cap B / A$. These results, shown in Table 1 (left), demonstrate that typically over 80% of the locations with increased diffusion also yield a high error of fit

Table 1. Dice coefficients between voxels A with high ADC (>0.6) and voxels B with high error of fit (>15) degrees.

Pig	$A \cap B / A \cup B$	$A \cap B / A$
Pig 2	.40	.80
Pig 4	.43	.89
Pig 5	.47	.76
Pig 6	.46	.87
Pig 7	.27	.94

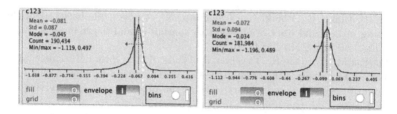

Fig. 4. Histograms of the c_{123} connection parameter over all voxels with low error of fit in an infarcted heart (left) and over all voxels in a healthy heart (right).

using our frame fitting method, due to the loss of geometric coherence of fiber orientations. However there are additional locations where fiber orientations are not smooth, typically at the linings of the heart wall, or near the edges of a collapsing and narrow right ventricle. Such regions are not picked up by the ADC or FA measures likely because there is no increase in collagen or loss in anisotropy there. As such, we hypothesize that these are regions where the fiber orientation is simply distinct from that of neighboring locations, i.e., it does not form a coherent pattern.

We also present histograms in Fig. 4 to compare the c_{123} connection parameter in the infarcted pig heart of Fig. 1, but restricted to locations where the error of fit is low, with the c_{123} parameter for the healthy heart. This connection parameter attains by far the largest values in healthy hearts, because it relates to the transmural turning of fibers from outer wall to inner wall. The histograms have very similar distributions and mean values in voxel units, suggesting that in regions away from the infarct, the fiber geometry remains similar to that of a healthy heart.

4   Conclusion

We have demonstrated the use of Cartan frame fitting to characterize collagenous fibrosis and to provide quantitative assessment of fiber coherence in the presence of structural heart disease, using high resolution DW imaging in infarcted porcine hearts. Although our Cartan frame fits were applied to a relatively small sample size of 5 diseased hearts and 1 healthy one, the results are consistent and the method holds promise for the measurement of fiber coherence in dense scar areas and more importantly in the BZ, where the substrate of lethal arrhythmia resides. In future work we plan to carry out this analysis using in vivo DW MR data, in an effort to integrate our frame fitting methods into clinical platforms for better differential diagnosis. We also hope to provide personalized estimates of fiber directions for use in mathematical models for in silico prediction of electro-mechanical function in hearts with infarcts.

References

1. Bayer, J., Blake, R., Plank, G., Trayanova, N.: A novel rule-based algorithm for assigning myocardial fiber orientation to computational heart models. Ann. Biomed. Eng. **40**(10), 2243–2254 (2012)
2. de Baker, J.M., Coronel, R., Tasseron, S., Wilde, A.A., Opthof, T., Janse, M.J., van Capelle, F.J., Becker, A.E., Jambroes, G.: Ventricular tachyrdia in the infarcted, langendorff-perfused human heart: role of the arrangement of surviving cardiac fibers. J. Am. Coll. Cardiol. **15**(7), 1594–1607 (1990)
3. Holmes, J., Yamashita, H., Waldman, L., Covell, J.: Scar remodeling and transmural deformation after infarction in the pig. Circulation **90**(1), 411–420 (1994)
4. Horowitz, A., Perl, M., Sideman, S.: Geodesics as a mechanically optimal fiber geometry for the left ventricle. Basic. Res. Cardiol. **88**(Suppl 2), 67–74 (1993)
5. McCormick, R.J., Musch, T.I., Bergman, B.C., Thomas, D.P.: Regional differences in LV collagen accumulation and mature cross-linking after myocardial infarction in rats. Am. J. Physiol. Heart Circulatory Physiol. **266**(1), H354–H359 (1994)
6. Peskin, C.S.: Fiber architecture of the left ventricular wall: an asymptotic analysis. Commun. Pure Appl. Math. **42**(1), 79–113 (1989)
7. Piuze, E., Sporring, J., Siddiqi, K.: Maurer-cartan forms for fields on surfaces: application to heart fiber geometry. IEEE Trans. Pattern Anal. Mach. Intell. **37**(12), 2492–2504 (2015)
8. Pop, M., Ghugre, N.R., Ramanan, V., Morikawa, L., Stanisz, G., Dick, A.J., Wright, G.A.: Quantification of fibrosis in infarcted swine hearts by ex vivo late gadolinium-enhancement and diffusion-weighted MRI methods. Phys. Med. Biol. **58**(15), 5009 (2013)
9. Savadjiev, P., Strijkers, G.J., Bakermans, A.J., Piuze, E., Zucker, S.W., Siddiqi, K.: Heart wall myofibers are arranged in minimal surfaces to optimize organ function. Proc. Natl. Acad. Sci. **109**(24), 9248–9253 (2012)
10. Streeter, D.D.: Gross morphology and fiber geometry of the heart. In: Berne, R.M., Sperelakis, N. (eds.) Handbook of Physiology, Section 2. The Heart, pp. 61–112. Williams and Wilkins, New York (1979)
11. Swynghedauw, B.: Molecular mechanisms of myocardial remodeling. Physiol. Rev. **79**(1), 215–262 (1999)
12. Ursell, P.C., Gardner, P.I., Albala, A., Fenoglio, J., Wit, A.L.: Structural and electrophysiological changes in the epicardial border zone of canine myocardial infarcts during infarct healing. Circ. Res. **56**(3), 436–451 (1985)
13. Wiest-Daesslé, N., Prima, S., Coupé, P., Morrissey, S.P., Barillot, C.: Rician noise removal by non-local means filtering for low signal-to-noise ratio MRI: applications to DT-MRI. In: Metaxas, D., Axel, L., Fichtinger, G., Székely, G. (eds.) MICCAI 2008. LNCS, vol. 5242, pp. 171–179. Springer, Heidelberg (2008). doi:10.1007/978-3-540-85990-1_21

14. Wu, E.X., Wu, Y., Nicholls, J.M., Wang, J., Liao, S., Zhu, S., Lau, C.-P., Tse, H.-F.: MR diffusion tensor imaging study of postinfarct myocardium structural remodeling in a porcine model. Magn. Reson. Med. **58**(4), 687–695 (2007)

15. Wu, M.-T., Su, M.-Y.M., Huang, Y.-L., Chiou, K.-R., Yang, P., Pan, H.-B., Reese, T.G., Wedeen, V.J., Tseng, W.-Y.I.: Sequential changes of myocardial microstructure in patients postmyocardial infarction by diffusion-tensor cardiac mr correlation with left ventricular structure and function. Circ. Cardiovasc. Imaging **2**(1), 32–40 (2009)

16. Zipes, D.P.: Epidemiology and mechanisms of sudden cardiac death. Can. J. Cardiol. **21**, 37A–40A (2005)

Standardised Framework to Study the Influence of Left Atrial RF Catheter Ablation Parameters on Permanent Lesion Formation

Marta Nuñez-Garcia[1(✉)], David Andreu[2], Marta Male[1], Francisco Alarcon[2], Lluís Mont[2], Constantine Butakoff[1], and Oscar Camara[1]

[1] PhySense, DTIC, Universitat Pompeu Fabra, Barcelona, Spain
`marta.nunez@upf.edu`
[2] Arrhythmia Section, Cardiology Department,
Thorax Institute, Hospital Clínic and IDIBAPS
(Institut d'Investigacions Biomèdiques August Pi i Sunyer), Barcelona, Spain

Abstract. Radiofrequency ablation is a common procedure to treat atrial fibrillation, where the objective is to electrically isolate some regions of the myocardium from others to avoid the transmission of abnormal electrical signals. This is done with a catheter by delivering an RF signal in the targeted regions. Ideally, the signal will create a permanent lesion that would prevent the reappearance of the abnormal electrical signals and therefore terminate AF. There are many parameters involved in the process and naturally in its success. In this paper we present a framework for comparing RF ablation related parameters such as power of the signal, contact force, temperature and impedance with permanent and effective lesion formation. In order to do that we propose to use a standardised unfold map that allows us to directly compare atria with different shapes at different time-points and with different types of information. We tested the method in 8 real cases showing that it facilitates the analysis and comparison of the ablation related parameters with the outcome of the procedure.

Keywords: Left atrium · Radiofrequency catheter ablation · Contact Force · Pulmonary vein isolation · Unfold map

1 Introduction

Atrial fibrillation (AF) triggers are mainly located inside pulmonary veins (PV) [9]. Radiofrequency (RF) PV isolation (PVI) is the most frequent procedure to treat AF [5] by electrically isolating the veins to avoid the transmission of the abnormal electrical signals. The procedure consists in delivering RF energy (typically 30–40 W, 500 kHz) over the tip of a therapy electrophysiology catheter during a certain time across the perimeter of the (typically) four PV. According to Ganesan et al. [7] the long-term success rate ranges from 53.1% with a singe procedure to almost 80% with multiple procedures.

© Springer International Publishing AG 2017
T. Mansi et al. (Eds.): STACOM 2016, LNCS 10124, pp. 96–105, 2017.
DOI: 10.1007/978-3-319-52718-5_11

One of the reasons for this low success rate is the incomplete isolation of the PV due to punctual ablation and the presence of gaps in the lesion (scar or fibrous tissue). Several authors [8,13], have investigated the influence of these anatomical gaps in the recurrence rate of AF. Clearly, incorrect RF ablation (e.g. when the catheter does not touch the LA wall) is a reason for incomplete PV isolation but also other involved parameters can favour the non formation of an effective lesion causing AF recurrence. Parameters related to the delivery of the RF energy such as power of the signal, contact force (CF) [14], temperature or impedance drop may play an important role.

The objective of this study is to investigate the influence of ablation-related parameters on the scar formation around the PVs assessed by a post ablation Late Gadolinium Enhancement (LGE) Cardiovascular Magnetic Resonance (CMR) study. Recent studies have reported the capability of identifying RF ablation lesions in the LA in a 3 months post ablation LGE-CMR study [12], and even to identify lesion gaps in the PV circumference ablation line [1,4]. The task is challenging due to several reasons: during the ablation parameters are recorded at discrete locations (points, coordinates) and a method is needed to merge the information about the LA shape (previously extracted to help guiding the catheter) and the recorded points; additionally, there is LA remodelling due to the ablation procedure and to AF itself [11] and therefore it is difficult to directly compare different atrial shapes; LA segmentation is complicated due to insufficient image resolution to capture thin atrial wall and the segmented LA shapes may appear even more different than they actually are due to segmentation errors.

Trying to overcome these complications several alternative representations of the LA have been proposed. For example, Karim et al. [10] implemented a surface flattening method where one of the clinical applications was to display and compare the unfolded electroanatomical map (endocardial voltage) obtained from mapping systems with the unfolded LGE-CMR map. However, the generated maps are patient-specific and the method does not allow direct comparison between different patients. Therefore, we propose to use the standardised unfold map of the LA defined in [16] that allows us to represent in the same reference system the LA tissue information obtained from the LGE-CMR study and the ablation parameters sampled during the procedure. Having this standard representation we can locally or globally correlate all the parameters involved in the ablation with the scar formation. In addition, we can directly compare results from different patients and investigate the existence of optimal values.

2 Method

The complete framework has four main stages, each of which is explained next. A complete scheme can be seen in Fig. 1.

1. Acquisition of RF-ablation Related Parameters.

In order to integrate the parameters of the RF ablation in a common space the first step is to obtain a representation of the LA shape. Previous to the

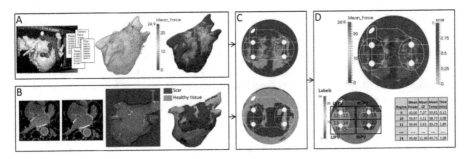

Fig. 1. Complete framework. A. Extraction of the pre-ablation atrial shape and projection of the RF-ablation related parameters (automatically recorded during the ablation and saved in text files (the numbers shown here are unimportant)). In the figure, contact force is shown. B. Extraction of the post-ablation atrial shape and LA wall tissue characterisation: binary classification into either scar or healthy tissue (gaps would be classified as healthy tissue). C. Standardised unfold map of the LA shapes. D. Regional analysis and comparison of the two standardised unfold maps. The upper disk shows the two maps superimposed and the table shows results from the numerical analysis per region (this is an example and the numbers are irrelevant). In the small disk it can be seen the regional division of the LA.

ablation procedure and with the aim of helping guiding the catheter all patients undergo an image study (Computed Tomography (CT) or CMR). The anatomical information is obtained by delineating the LA shape followed by some pre-process (smooth and mesh correction basically) in order to eliminate artefacts due to imaging. This pre-process reduces the potential differences between the two acquisition methods used. During the intervention the mesh is imported into the navigation system and aligned with the current view by rigid registration (rotation and translation). Using the registration matrix it is possible to realign the original mesh and the recorded points afterwards. In the proposed framework this alignment is done by calculating the inverse transformation and applying it to the ablation-related points.

During the ablation the following parameters are saved into the system with a sampling period of 17 ms: position of the catheter tip, power, contact force, temperature and impedance. All this information is projected onto the LA mesh as follows: for each ablation-related sample we find its closest point (vertex) in the mesh. It is noticeable that several ablation-related points may lie on the same LA mesh point. In that situation information is accumulated in the corresponding vertex. Accordingly, vertices of the LA mesh without projected ablation-related points have an assigned value of 0 and are not used in the numerical analysis. The output of this stage is a LA mesh showing the pre-ablation LA anatomy with that information projected (see Fig. 1A).

2. Tissue Characterization of the Post Ablated LA.

Delayed-enhancement CMR images of patients that underwent ablation therapy are typically acquired some months after the procedure in order to assess its success. The regular clinical practice at Hospital Clínic (Barcelona) is to perform the CMR study 3 months after the ablation. From these images, the shape of the LA is extracted by manual segmentation of the LA wall. Binary tissue classification (scar or healthy) is then performed according to the method presented in [3]: Local Image Intensity Ratio (IIR) is calculated as the ratio between the pixel and the mean blood pool intensities. The authors established thresholds based on healthy volunteers and post-ablation patients: an $IIR \leq 1.20$ identifies normal atrial tissue, and an $IIR > 1.32$ identifies dense scarring (see Fig. 1B).

3. Standardised Unfold Map (SUM).

A standardised unfold map (SUM) was proposed in [16] and its main steps are:

1. Mesh standardisation: the PVs and the left atrial appendage (LAA) are semi-automatically clipped. The algorithm requires to manually place a seed close to the ending point of each PV and the LAA. After that, the PVs and LAA are automatically clipped at a distance of the ostium that can be set by the user. Also the mitral valve (MV) is automatically clipped using the information of the placed seeds. We decided to clip the LAA because it is not directly related to PVI. It is important to note that it can extremely vary between different subjects and therefore with that decision we minimise its influence in the following steps.
2. Surface registration of the template where the regions were defined to the standardised atrium resulting from the previous step. This is done by a non-rigid registration based on currents [6] after an initial affine registration.
3. Projection of the registered template to a disk: the MV is mapped to the boundary of the disk and the PV and LAA holes are mapped to predefined holes within the disk.

The resulting disk is a parcellated 2D standard representation of the LA that permits the comparison of the pre- and post-ablated atria that, it is important to remember, have different shapes. In addition, the parcellation of the disk permits performing regional analysis. Finally, representing atria in a 2D map favours fast interpretability and visualisation of the data.

4. Analysis and Comparison of the Ablation and Scar SUMs.

The output of the previous step is a pair of SUMs for each patient: one with ablation-related parameters (i.e. power, contact force, temperature and impedance) and the other one with binary scar segmentation. Let us name these maps *ablation-SUM* and *scar-SUM*. For comparing these two maps we propose the following:

1. Use the parcellation provided by the SUM to evaluate RF-ablation related parameters in each region of the *ablation-SUM*. As we are interested in evaluating the success of PVI we focus in regions representing the surroundings of

each PV. For each vein, its surroundings are divided in four quadrants, thus 16 regions are analysed. We compute the mean and total values of power, contact force and temperature in each SUM region.

2. Localise gaps in the *scar-SUM*. For doing this we follow a strategy similar to the one we recently presented in [8]: we define the *isolating path* as the scar-path that encircles a PV with the minimum amount of gap. We then identify the regions of the SUM where a gap is present. In this study we do not consider the relative amount of gap, only if there is a gap or not. If the gap is less than 10% of the isolating path is ignored.

3. Correlate the information about the gaps (yes/no) with the ablation parameters in all regions: mean and total power, contact force and temperature. With regard to the impedance it is interesting to analyse the impedance drop. In this initial version of the framework we project all the samples to the LA mesh loosing the time reference. We need to take into account the particular temporal instant in order to be able of analysing impedance drops. This could be done complementing the framework adding temporal information but it was left to future work.

Ultimate objective is then to find differences regarding the parameters between regions with and without gaps.

3   Experiments and Results

We applied the proposed method to 8 real cases. The RF catheter used was the Thermocool SmartTouch[1] and the ablation information was acquired with CARTO (See footnote 1). Anatomical information was incorporated from pre-interventional CT or CMR images and the LA shape was extracted from the DICOM images using a research software (ADAS[2]) or CartoMERGE in the case of CT images. The number of ablation-related samples in our data was $98,821 \pm 3,302$ samples. As mentioned before the sampling rate for automatically acquiring these samples was 17 ms, which explains the high number of recorded points. On the other hand, regarding the *scar-SUM*, manual segmentations of the LA wall surface were extracted also using tha ADAS software and tissue classification was performed according to [3] as explained in Sect. 2. For the generation of the SUMs we decided to keep a PV and LAA length of 3 mm in all the cases. The complete framework (pre-processing, mapping and post-processing) was coded in Python using the VTK library. We also used reMESH [2] for correcting mesh imperfections.

Figure 2 and Table 1 show the SUMs generated for one patient and its numerical analysis. The power of the signal was not studied since the recommended power (40 W) was used for all cases. Nevertheless, we found that the mean value is slightly inferior because there are growing and decreasing slopes when passing from 0 W to 40 W and vice versa. With relation to the temperature it can be seen that it is

---

[1] Biosense Webster Inc, Diamond Bar, CA.

[2] ADAS, Galgo Medical SL. Barcelona, Spain.

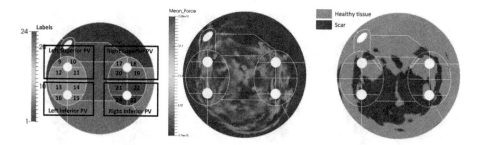

Fig. 2. Example of the 2 SUMs generated for one patient. From left to right: template with region labels; *ablation-SUM* showing in this case the information about contact force; *scar-SUM* showing the segmented scar (magenta) and the detected gaps (yellow). (Color figure online)

Table 1. Some results from the numerical analysis of the example in Fig. 2.

Region	Mean power (W)	Mean contact force (g)	Mean temperature (°C)	Mean time (min)	Gap?
9	37,56	5,29	41,98	2,60	Too small
10	39,32	3,85	42,14	5,05	**Yes**
11	34,99	9,18	41,37	1,12	**Yes**
12	38,49	7,40	41,53	2,41	No
13	39,33	6,10	42,02	0,36	No
14	36,79	3,61	42,74	1,33	No
15	36,17	5,64	41,30	2,17	No
16	36,65	4,87	40,01	0,17	No
17	37,56	4,73	41,57	1,12	**Yes**
18	39,93	6,42	42,12	1,28	No
19	38,66	7,36	41,49	3,25	No
20	35,83	6,76	41,68	3,15	**Yes**
21	39,96	4,22	42,41	2,23	No
22	38,77	6,87	41,92	2,17	No
23	35,13	9,46	40,16	1,37	No
24	39,88	4,47	42,45	0,33	No

Table 2. Numerical analysis results: comparison between regions with and without gap. Shown is the mean ± standard error of power, contact force, temperature, number of CARTO samples and time.

	Power (W)	Force (g)	Temperature (°C)	# CARTO samples	Time (min)
No gap	34.74 ± 1.88	7.82 ± 1.00	39.55 ± 0.94	5035.09 ± 1566.39	1.43 ± 0.44
Gap	34.95 ± 1.34	8.01 ± 0.80	39.35 ± 0.67	7550.80 ± 1857.57	2.14 ± 0.53

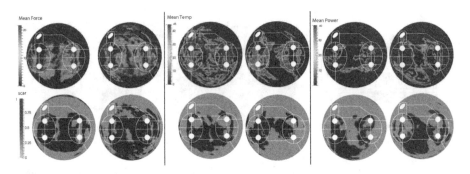

Fig. 3. Examples of pair of SUMs generated: the first row shows *ablation-SUM* and the second row their corresponding *scar-SUM* (each column is a different patient). Regarding the ablation-SUMs examples of contact force, temperature and power are shown.

significantly lower than the typically target temperature (i.e. 50–55 °C). This is due to the fact that the ablation was done with an irrigated catheter (in order to induce a deeper lesion) which is a type of cooled tip ablation [15,17].

In the example shown in Fig. 2, it can be observed that there are two gaps: one in the left superior PV (LSPV) and the other one in the right superior PV (RSPV). Results in Table 1 suggest that the gap in region 10 can be due to low CF even though the ablation time is quite high. We could also hypothesise that the gap in region 11 corresponds to an area insufficiently ablated (see *ablation-SUM* in that region). If we compare regions 17 and 18 we can see that the two regions were ablated during a similar period of time but in region 17 the mean CF and mean power were lower than in region 18. This fact could explain why we see a gap in region 17 and not in region 18. Likewise, if we compare regions 19 and 20 that were also ablated during a similar period of time, we observe again that the mean CF and mean power are lower in the region where there is a gap (20). However, we observe that in other regions good scar patterns were obtained with lower CF, power and in less time. Examples of efficient ablations can be seen in regions 13, 16 and 18 where a good scar pattern was created in a short period of time (see Fig. 2).

We compared the numerical analysis of all patients trying to find common patterns relating the parameters and the presence or absence of anatomical gaps but statistically significant differences were not found (see Table 2). We also analysed the influence of the ablation time: we investigated whether it is more effective to ablate during a shorter period of time with a higher contact force or with lower contact force during a longer period of time but there was not any consistent pattern. Even more, unexpectedly, we found that regions with gaps were ablated (in average) much time and with a higher CF (Fig. 3).

4 Discussion and Conclusions

We have presented a framework to analyse the influence of RF-ablation parameters in the formation of a permanent lesion that would, ideally, terminate AF. For that, we decided to use a standardised unfold map that permits directly compare atria with different shapes and with different kind of information. Our aim was to identify optimal values of the parameters but we did not find clear thresholds from our experiments. Some potential reasons are: (1) The dataset is too small for extracting well founded conclusions; (2) The LA wall is very thin and its segmentation is complicated: there are segmentation errors that can affect the results; (3) Patients with AF may have natural fibrosis (not induced by the ablation) that would be classified as scar in the tissue classification process. It would be convenient to perform tissue classification previous to the RF-ablation in order to be able to differentiate between natural and ablation induced fibrosis. For this study we did not have access to the pre-ablation images but we plan to enrich the method by including this information in the future; (4) The objective during the ablation is to have as less gaps as possible and therefore in the data there are not many of them.

For future work we plan to have access to a bigger dataset and improve the segmentation method used. We also plan to automatically analyse the amount of gap in each of the SUM regions and not only its presence or absence. Similarly to what was done in [8], we will investigate if there is correlation between the parameters and a quantitative measure describing the amount of gap in each region.

Acknowledgements. This work was partially supported by the EU FP7 for research, technological development and demonstration under grant agreement VP2HF (no 611823) and by the Spanish Ministry of Economy and Competitiveness (DPI2015-71640-R). The authors would like to thank Catalina Tobon-Gomez, Steven E. Williams and M. Henry Chubb for their valuable help.

References

1. Andreu, D., Gomez-Pulido, F., Calvo, M., Carlosena-Remírez, A., Bisbal, F., Borràs, R., Benito, E., Guasch, E., Prat-Gonzalez, S., Perea, R.J., et al.: Contact force threshold for permanent lesion formation in atrial fibrillation ablation: a cardiac magnetic resonance-based study to detect ablation gaps. Heart Rhythm **13**(1), 37–45 (2016)
2. Attene, M., Falcidieno, B.: Remesh: an interactive environment to edit and repair triangle meshes. In: IEEE International Conference on Shape Modeling and Applications, p. 41 (2006)
3. Benito, E., Carlosena-Remírez, A., Guasch, E., Prat-Gonzalez, S., Perea, R.J., Figueras, R., Borràs, R., Andreu, D., Arbelo, E., Tolosana, J.M., Bisbal, F., Berruezo, A., Brugada, J., Mont, L.: Left atrial fibrosis quantification by late gadolinium enhancement magnetic resonance: a new method to standardize the thresholds for reproducibility. Europace. Epub ahead of print (2016)

4. Bisbal, F., Guiu, E., Cabanas-Grandío, P., Berruezo, A., Prat-Gonzalez, S., Vidal, B., Garrido, C., Andreu, D., Fernandez-Armenta, J., Tolosana, J.M., et al.: Cmr-guided approach to localize and ablate gaps in repeat af ablation procedure. JACC: Cardiovasc. Imaging **7**(7), 653–663 (2014)
5. Calkins, H., Kuck, K.H., Cappato, R., Brugada, J., Camm, A.J., Chen, S.A., Crijns, H.J., Damiano, R.J., Davies, D.W., DiMarco, J., et al.: 2012 HRS/EHRA/ECAS expert consensus statement on catheter and surgical ablation of atrial fibrillation: recommendations for patient selection, procedural techniques, patient management and follow-up, definitions, endpoints, and research trial design. Europace **14**(4), 528–606 (2012)
6. Durrleman, S., Prastawa, M., Charon, N., Korenberg, J.R., Joshi, S., Gerig, G., Trouvé, A.: Morphometry of anatomical shape complexes with dense deformations and sparse parameters. NeuroImage **101**, 35–49 (2014)
7. Ganesan, A.N., Shipp, N.J., Brooks, A.G., Kuklik, P., Lau, D.H., Lim, H.S., Sullivan, T., Roberts-Thomson, K.C., Sanders, P.: Long-term outcomes of catheter ablation of atrial fibrillation: a systematic review and meta-analysis. J. Am. Heart Assoc. **2**(2), e004549 (2013)
8. Nuñez Garcia, M., Tobon-Gomez, C., Rhode, K., Bijnens, B., Camara, O., Butakoff, C.: Quantification of gaps in ablation lesions around the pulmonary veins in delayed enhancement MRI. In: van Assen, H., Bovendeerd, P., Delhaas, T. (eds.) FIMH 2015. LNCS, vol. 9126, pp. 215–222. Springer, Heidelberg (2015). doi:10.1007/978-3-319-20309-6_25
9. Haissaguerre, M., Jaïs, P., Shah, D.C., Takahashi, A., Hocini, M., Quiniou, G., Garrigue, S., Le Mouroux, A., Le Métayer, P., Clémenty, J.: Spontaneous initiation of atrial fibrillation by ectopic beats originating in the pulmonary veins. New Engl. J. Med. **339**(10), 659–666 (1998)
10. Karim, R., Ma, Y., Jang, M., Housden, R.J., Williams, S.E., Chen, Z., Ataollahi, A., Althoefer, K., Rinaldi, C.A., Razavi, R., et al.: Surface flattening of the human left atrium and proof-of-concept clinical applications. Comput. Med. Imaging Graph. **38**(4), 251–266 (2014)
11. Kuppahally, S.S., Akoum, N., Badger, T.J., Burgon, N.S., Haslam, T., Kholmovski, E., Macleod, R., McGann, C., Marrouche, N.F.: Echocardiographic left atrial reverse remodeling after catheter ablation of atrial fibrillation is predicted by pre-ablation delayed enhancement of left atrium by magnetic resonance imaging. Am. Heart J. **160**(5), 877–884 (2010)
12. McGann, C., Kholmovski, E., Blauer, J., Vijayakumar, S., Haslam, T., Cates, J., DiBella, E., Burgon, N., Wilson, B., Alexander, A., et al.: Dark regions of no-reflow on late gadolinium enhancement magnetic resonance imaging result in scar formation after atrial fibrillation ablation. J. Am. Coll. Cardiol. **58**(2), 177–185 (2011)
13. Peters, D.C., Wylie, J.V., Hauser, T.H., Nezafat, R., Han, Y., Woo, J.J., Taclas, J., Kissinger, K.V., Goddu, B., Josephson, M.E., et al.: Recurrence of atrial fibrillation correlates with the extent of post-procedural late gadolinium enhancement: a pilot study. JACC: Cardiovasc. Imaging **2**(3), 308–316 (2009)
14. Shurrab, M., Di Biase, L., Briceno, D.F., Kaoutskaia, A., Haj-Yahia, S., Newman, D., Lashevsky, I., Nakagawa, H., Crystal, E.: Impact of contact force technology on atrial fibrillation ablation: a meta-analysis. J. Am. Heart Assoc. **4**(9), e002476 (2015)
15. Thomas, S.P., Aggarwal, G., Boyd, A.C., Jin, Y., Ross, D.L.: A comparison of open irrigated and non-irrigated tip catheter ablation for pulmonary vein isolation. Europace **6**(4), 330–335 (2004)

16. Tobon-Gomez, C., Zuluaga, M.A., Chubb, H., Williams, S.E., Butakoff, C., Karim, R., Camara, O., Ourselin, S., Rhode, K.: Standardised unfold map of the left atrium: regional definition for multimodal image analysis. J. Cardiovasc. Magn. Reson. **17**(1), 1 (2015)

17. Yamane, T., Jaïs, P., Shah, D.C., Hocini, M., Peng, J.T., Deisenhofer, I., Clémenty, J., Haïssaguerre, M.: Efficacy and safety of an irrigated-tip catheter for the ablation of accessory pathways resistant to conventional radiofrequency ablation. Circulation **102**(21), 2565–2568 (2000)

From CMR Image to Patient-Specific Simulation and Population-Based Analysis: Tutorial for an Openly Available Image-Processing Pipeline

Maciej Marciniak[1]([✉]), Hermenegild Arevalo[1], Jacob Tfelt-Hansen[2],
Thomas Jespersen[3], Reza Jabbari[2], Charlotte Glinge[2], Kiril A. Ahtarovski[2],
Niels Vejlstrup[2], Thomas Engstrom[2], Mary M. Maleckar[1],
and Kristin McLeod[1,4]

[1] Cardiac Modelling Department, Simula Research Laboratory, Oslo, Norway
maciej.mar92@gmail.com
[2] Department of Cardiology, Rigshospitalet, Copenhagen, Denmark
[3] Department of Biomedical Sciences, University of Copenhagen,
Copenhagen, Denmark
[4] Centre for Cardiological Innovation, Oslo, Norway

Abstract. Cardiac magnetic resonance (CMR) imaging is becoming a routine diagnostic and therapy planning tool for some cardiovascular diseases. It is still challenging to properly analyse the acquired data, and the currently available measures do not exploit the rich characteristics of that data. Advanced analysis and modelling techniques are increasingly used to extract additional information from the images, in order to define metrics describing disease manifestations and to quantitatively compare patients. Many techniques share a common bottleneck caused by the image processing required to segment the images and convert the segmentation to a usable computational domain for analysis/modelling. To address this, we present a comprehensive pipeline to go from CMR images to computational bi-ventricle meshes. The latter can be used for biophysical simulations or statistical shape analysis. The provided tutorial describes each step and the proposed pipeline, which makes use of tools that are available open-source. The pipeline was applied to a data-set of myocardial infarction patients, from late gadolinium enhanced CMR images, to analyse and compare structure in these patients. Examples of applications present the use of the output of the pipeline for patient-specific biophysical simulations and population-based statistical shape analysis.

1 Introduction

Patient-specific simulations and population-based modelling are becoming increasingly popular in analyzing cardiac disease to extract important information about causes of arrhythmogenic or mechanical dysfunctions, and remodelling that occurs as a result of a disease. Such computational models have proven useful, for example, in detecting re-entry sites for arrhythmias [1] and to quantify structural abnormalities [2].

© Springer International Publishing AG 2017
T. Mansi et al. (Eds.): STACOM 2016, LNCS 10124, pp. 106–117, 2017.
DOI: 10.1007/978-3-319-52718-5_12

Computational patient-specific simulation requires segmentation of the anatomy from imaging. In the case of population-based modelling, pre-alignment of all subjects to a common frame is required, to remove differences in pose. For electrophysiology simulations of ischemic heart disease, segmentation of the scar or ischemic regions has to be performed. These regions are important pre-cursors in many arrhythmic disorders. Going from medical images to computational geometries can be time-consuming, laborious and prone to human error.

Since CMR imaging enables tissue characterisation through late gadolinium enhancement (LGE) imaging, the use of LGE is becoming increasingly popular. Due to the lack of openly available and automated tools, we developed a pipeline from LGE images to computational geometries that makes use of a freely available and widely used cardiac image segmentation software tool (Segment, Medviso). The proposed pipeline processes the segmentation to remove slice misalignment, to align all segmented data to a common reference (for comparative analysis and statistical shape modelling), and to build three-dimensional (3D) volumetric models of the geometry and scar regions (for electrophysiological simulation). A tutorial provides detailed steps of the proposed open-source pipeline and potential uses of the pipeline are described in our examples applied to myocardial infarction patients. 3D model generation and the techniques used to process the scar information are detailed in Sects. 2 and 3.

2   Bi-ventricle and Scar Segmentation

In the present work, 3D segmentation of the left and right ventricular endocardium, bi-ventricular epicardium, and scar (infarct) region from LGE images (in the end-diastolic phase) is performed. For this task, Segment; a software package for medical image analysis from Medviso [3], is used. A screenshot showing the functionality of Segment is given in Fig. 1. A full tutorial describing how to perform segmentation in Segment is provided on their website[1].

Ventricle segmentation is accomplished by either manually or automatically drawing contours around the endocardium and epicardium surfaces of both ventricles on each two-dimensional (2D) image slice. Automatic segmentation within Segment is performed using level-set and deformable contour algorithms [4]. The algorithm creates both endo- and epicardial borders for the left ventricle (LV), which the user can adjust if necessary. Because of the complexity in shape of the right ventricle (RV), segmentation in Segment is performed semi-manually. In proposed pipeline, the tool for segmentation of the right ventricle epicardium is used to define the bi-ventricular epicardium. Segmentation is performed up to the last basal slice before the valve plane, defined as the first slice which divides into inlet and outlet of either ventricle. The bi-ventricular epicardium is required to generate a volumetric mesh for biophysical simulations. Sets of data points, which describe both epi- and endocardial borders of the ventricles, are saved from the image itself for each slice of the LGE stack.

---

[1] www.medviso.com.

The scar region is automatically delineated with an algorithm that also incorporates partial volume effects by weighting the infarct volume by pixel intensity [5]. The underlying algorithm for finding infarct is based on Expectation Maximization (EM algorithm). It is necessary to perform segmentation of the left ventricle first, as the ischemic regions are found between the endo- and epicardium of the LV. The method for computing scar in Segment is described in [6].

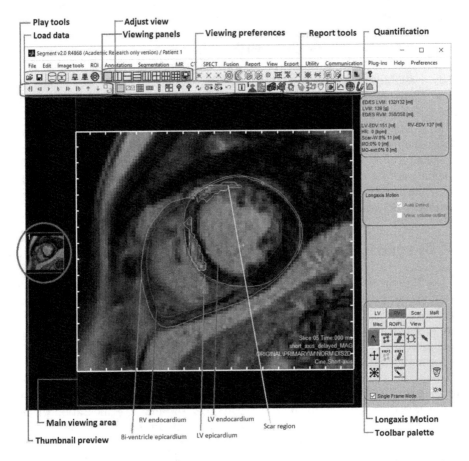

Fig. 1. Annotated screenshot of the Segment user interface with highlighted main units, which shows functionality of the tool. Segmented ventricles with defined scar regions can be seen in the main viewing area.

3   Automatic Pre-processing Pipeline

3.1   3D Model Generation

From the slice-wise segmentation, a point-cloud defining the boundary (surface) points on each slice is exported. Acquired point-clouds are then processed in order to locate them in the same space [6]. Breath-hold artefact correction is achieved through calculating linear least square estimation of the vertical axis of the LV, according to the 2D barycenters of each slice. The barycenter of a given slice is then aligned to the slice above and the slice below. This is applied to point-clouds corresponding to both ventricles as well as to the scar regions.

Performing statistical shape analysis on meshes created in further steps requires both ventricles of every subject to be in the same physical space (i.e. to be rigidly aligned). Therefore, spatial alignment is performed to shift and rotate all subjects to a reference subject. This is necessary to reduce the bias in construction of the mean and to focus on calculating differences in the anatomy instead of position and/or orientation of given subjects. Alignment of all subjects is performed by taking the 3D barycenter of each ventricle from the endocardial point-clouds, and then a line-segment joining the LV and RV barycenters is computed. The rigid transformation from the line-segment of each subject to the line-segment of the arbitrarily chosen reference subject is computed. All point-clouds are then transformed by the computed line-segment transformation to align all 3D point-clouds. Translation parameters are based on the difference in positions of the barycenters in 3D space. Rotation is performed about the Z axis with angle θ defined as (Eq. 1)

$$\theta = cos^{-1} \left(\frac{u \cdot v}{||u|| \cdot ||v||} \right) \tag{1}$$

with u and v being vectors joining the line segments. This yields the following rotation matrix (Eq. 2)

$$R_Z(\theta) = \begin{bmatrix} cos\theta & -sin\theta & 0 \\ sin\theta & cos\theta & 0 \\ 0 & 0 & 1 \end{bmatrix} \tag{2}$$

Once all patients are aligned to a common space, the volumetric 3D tetrahedral meshes are generated by combining the RV endocardium with the LV endo- and epicardium, and the bi-ventricular epicardium.

3.2 Scar Post-processing

A binary image of scar regions is used to calculate coordinates of scar points in 3D. For each subject, the scar regions are defined with a 3D boolean array, and are transformed along with the ventricular segmentation (slice correction and pairwise alignment). In order to retrieve the coordinates in the same space as the segmented and aligned ventricles, indices of the positions with boolean 'one' are found. These indices correspond to the X and Y position of the scar regions in each slice. Obtained coordinates are then adjusted to the image resolution. The third (Z) coordinate is found by inserting the voxel depth for each slice, equal to the gap between slices in the ventricles plus the slice thickness. The point-cloud is then shifted along the Z axis, to the location of the left ventricle.

Obtained point-clouds (defining the scar/ischemic zone) are processed in order to create a proper, uniform volume of the scar on which further analysis can be performed. This scar volume must also be projected to the ventricular volumetric space, to keep it in the correct location. For this purpose, several image processing tools have been applied to the scar data sets (see Fig. 2) to:

- Eliminate outliers
- Resample voxels to be isotropic
- Smooth
- Calculate iso-contours

The first step in the processing pipeline is performed to remove noise in the scar image using a median image filter, which eliminates non-physiological outliers. By applying the filter, every pixel/data point is replaced with the median of its neighbours. The value of the radius, defining the furthest neighbour of the pixel/data point in each direction, can be selected depending on the desired level of noise reduction.

The second step is to account for the large inter-slice spacing in the acquired images, which may result in loss of important information encoded in the third dimension (along the Z axis). In order to make the images useful for further steps of image analysis, re-sampling of the data-set is conducted. Resampling of the voxel size in the Z direction is performed to obtain voxel sizes equal to the X and Y directions (which are equal). This results in an isotropic 3D image, which provides more insights and information in the 3D space than rigid connection of slices. Thirdly, a Gaussian smoothing to remove the staircase-effect in the images is performed.

Finally, the iso-contours are calculated to allow for visual analysis. This is essentially achieved by extracting the surface of the scar. The used filter defines the borders of an object and uses them to create a 3D mesh. The extracted surface is surrounding the pixels that define the scar region. The created pipeline is summarized in Fig. 2.

3.3   Implementation

As mentioned in Sect. 2, ventricular and scar segmentation was performed using Segment, a software package for medical image analysis from Medviso (FDA approved), freely available for research purposes. A licensed version is available for clinical use. The software not only allows segmentation with an easy-to-use interface, but also provides additional tools such as 3D visualisation of the obtained model, calculated volumes of both ventricles, and scar volume.

The described pre-processing pipeline steps were written in MATLAB (version R2015b). Point-clouds containing data describing the scar regions were saved as Insight Segmentation and Registration Toolkit (ITK)[2] .mhd images using the

---

[2] http://www.itk.org.

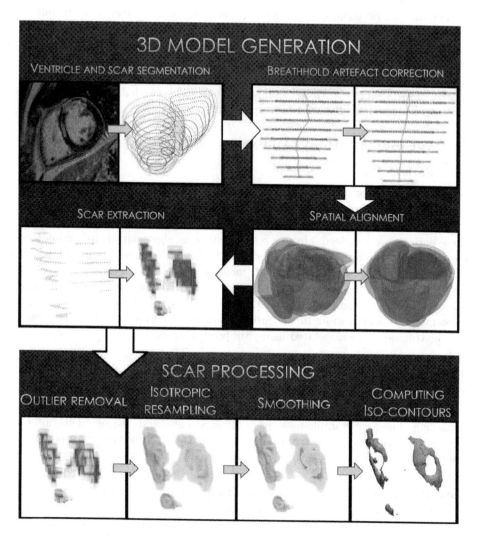

Fig. 2. The presented pipeline to go from a LGE image to point-clouds describing the endocardial surfaces of the left and right ventricles, the bi-ventricular epicardium, and scar regions (*ventricle and scar segmentation*), then to correct of slice misalignment caused by breath-holding (*breathhold artefact correction*), then to align subjects spatially to shift and rotate all subjects to a common space (*spatial alignment*), then to compute 3D scar volumes from the scar (ischemic) segmentation (*scar extraction*) and finally to post-processing of scar, which eliminates the outliers, and creates a 3D mesh (*scar processing*).

Medical Image Processing Toolbox[3]. The volumetric mesh generation is performed using Gmsh[4].

For the scar processing pipeline, the (ITK) was used which is an open-source, cross-platform system. Filters used for isotropic resampling, smoothing, and computing contours were written based on open-source examples[5]. Filtering was performed with shell script. Final results were visualised using Paraview from Kitware[6]. All codes used in this work are available open-source on Github repository[7]. Conversion of the Matlab code to python will be added in the near future to provide a pipeline that uses only open-source software.

4   Scar and Anatomy Analysis

4.1   Patient Data

The patient data used to develop the presented pipeline comes from an ongoing study in Denmark on genetic causes to ventricular arrhythmia in patients during first ST- elevation myocardial infarction (GEVAMI) [7]. LGE CMR images for these patients were collected from a retrospective database within approximately four weeks post-infarction period. A data-set of 8 patients, with varying extent of myocardial infarction, was studied: mean age $\pm$ standard deviation (years) $=59 \pm 9$. The final meshes for the two patients with the most significant ischemia are shown in Fig. 3, compared with 3D models of the segmentation from Segment. Slice misalignment, visible in 3D models, has been corrected for all patients. Infarct volumes were calculated using Simpsons rule [8].

4.2   Applications of the Presented Pipeline

To show how the presented pipeline can be used in practice, two examples are briefly described; one for patient-specific analysis and one for population-based modelling. The first example uses the volumetric mesh and scar segmentation to perform patient-specific electrophysiology simulation. The second example used the aligned surfaces to perform population-based statistical shape analysis.

Patient-Specific Electrophysiology Simulation: The presented pipeline was used to extract full 3D heart models with tissue characterisation (healthy/ischemic) for electrophysiology simulations on the MI patient data-set. A mono-domain electrophysiology model was used, modelling ischemic regions as having reduced conductivity, as described in [9]. An example of the electrophysiology solution for one of these patients is shown in Fig. 4. The electrophysiology simulations were run using the CARP software[8] (licensed software).

---

[3] www.mathworks.com/matlabcentral/fileexchange/41594-medical-image-processing-toolbox.

[4] http://gmsh.info.

[5] https://itk.org/Doxygen/html/examples.html.

[6] http://www.paraview.org.

[7] https://github.com/MAP-MD/Cardiac/tree/Cmr2Mesh.

[8] https://carp.medunigraz.at.

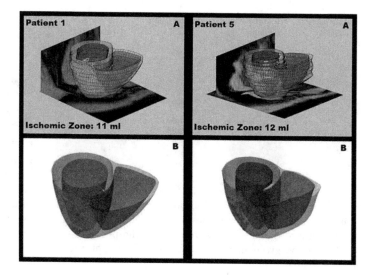

Fig. 3. The final meshes acquired with the pipeline in row B shown against the 3D model of the segmentation from Segment in row A. Presented patients have the greatest extent of ischemic zone.

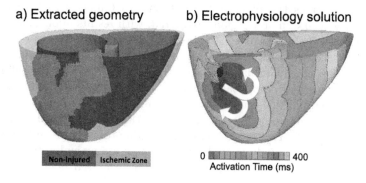

Fig. 4. (a) Example of a 3D heart model and tissue characterisation for one patient and (b) corresponding electrophysiology solution showing a reentrant circuit. Fiber directions were generated and integrated into the models using a rule-based algorithm.

Population-Based Ventricular Shape Analysis: Statistical shape analysis was applied to 8 patients to compute the most common shape features in the population (i.e. the shape modes). The ventricular surfaces were extracted and aligned using the presented pipeline. Principal component analysis (PCA) was used to compute the shape modes, following the methods described in [10]. Four shapes (modes) captured 90% of the shape variance in the population (see Fig. 5). The methods used to perform the statistical shape analysis are available open-source[9].

---

[9] www.deformetrica.com.

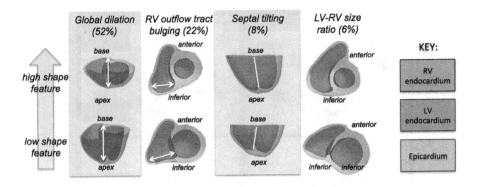

Fig. 5. The first four PCA shape modes (accounting for 90% of the shape variability in the population) are shown from low values (−2 standard deviations, bottom row), to high values (+2 standard deviations, top row), with the percentage of shape variance described by each shape given in brackets. Arrows highlight the important regions where changes are visible.

5 Discussion

This study describes the pipeline to go from CMR images to bi-ventricular meshes with scar and infarct regions extracted, with results applicable for both simulations and analysis. There have been a number of methods proposed for segmentation, scar extraction, image processing, and mesh generation, but only some of them are openly available. The tools used in the proposed pipeline were chosen for their usability, applicability, and availability. Our objective is not to create the optimal pipeline (given that gold standards do not exist and applications are varied), but rather to create a pipeline that could be easily adapted to other segmentation/scar extraction/mesh generation tools, and easily applicable to other modelling and analysis applications. There are many limitations to the currently available tools and methods, which are discussed below and will be addressed in future releases.

Tissue Characterisation: In the created pipeline, LGE was used for locating ischemic regions. It was considered in this study because despite its limitations and occurring variability of signal-to-noise ratio, LGE is still the most commonly used biomarker for tissue characterisation among clinicians. A different approach, such as T1 mapping, could be used for accurate in-vivo identification of fibrosis as an alternative, but is not widely used in clinical practice for scar quantification. More robust tools for scar detection are continuously being developed (e.g. those submitted to the 2012 STACOM challenge[10]) and might be of higher accuracy and wider use in the future.

Segmentation Method: Segmentation was performed using Segment, which was chosen for the presented pipeline due to the accessibility and easy-to-use inter-

---

[10] http://stacom.cardiacatlas.org/ventricular-infarction-challenge/.

face. What's more, it contains all the information needed to calculate the volumes of the scar and both ventricles, show weighted infarct transmurality, and visualise the pre-processed model. These utilities, contained in one software tool, comply with the requirements for full pipeline generation. The daily download rate of Segment is 5–6 downloads (including upgrades), with the number of unique new users per year reaching around 1500 (those that use unique email addresses). In addition, 17 clinical hospitals around the world use the commercial version of Segment (Segment CMR). To date, there are close to 600 journal publications that reference Segment. Therefore, it is a widely used tool and because it is continually improved with new methods as they become available, it will likely continue to be used for both research and clinical purposes. Potential expansion would include choosing different segmentation algorithms, such as those proposed in the STACOM 2011 challenge[11]. Furthermore, other open-source tools, such as Slicer[12], could have been used for segmentation and will be investigated. The proposed pipeline was applied to LGE images, but in the case where tissue classification is not required, the same pipeline could be applied e.g. to cine CMR images or T1 images.

Segmentation Area: In this study, valve segmentation is omitted due to the nature of exemplary applications. In general, statistical shape analysis and patient-specific electrophysiology simulations are conducted on computational ventricle models segmented from the frame below the valve plane. In future studies, valve modelling will be included using methods such as the one described in [11] to further increase the usability, provided that such tools become openly available.

Alignment and Correction: Slice correction and spatial alignment were both performed rigidly (i.e. no stretch or shear). Slice misalignment is not necessarily a rigid translation of the image slice, and could indeed include non-rigid transformation depending on the how consistently the patient held their breath for each scan. For simplicity, only rigid translation was considered in this pipeline, i.e. by calculating the vector joining the barycentre of each ventricle. Other rigid alignment techniques that consider the full geometry could be used, such as the robust point-set registration algorithm using Gaussian Mixture Models[13].

Image Processing Tool: In order to process the scar images, filter them, and compute contours, ITK was used. ITK is a cross-platform, open-source tool, which provides great functionality. Moreover, it is well documented and numerous examples of use are published on the official website. Filters and functions are constantly in development and added by independent users. ITK is the most commonly used tool for processing medical images, which was the main criterion for the choice of software in this study. Other tools for computational mesh

---

[11] http://www.cardiacatlas.org/challenges/lv-segmentation-challenge/.

[12] https://www.slicer.org.

[13] https://github.com/bing-jian/gmmreg.

generation, such as CGAL[14] or iso2mesh[15] could have been used as well and can be easily adopted in lieu of the tools used in the proposed pipeline.

Applications: Two potential applications were described: patient-specific biophysical simulation and population-based statistical shape analysis. The former is conducted with CARP software, which is only available under license. Although the purpose of describing this simulation was to show the applicability of the output of the pipeline, it is worth mentioning that open source tools, such as Fenics[16], ECGSim[17], Chaste[18] or CellML[19], or different methods [12] could be used for similar simulations. In addition, other statistical shape analyses could be applied to the computational ventricle meshes, for example those applied to the STACOM 2015 challenge[20].

6   Conclusion

A full pipeline from LGE CMR images to aligned computational surface meshes for population-based modelling or volumetric meshes with scar information for patient-specific biophysical simulations is presented. The pipeline includes steps to correct for breath-hold misalignment common in CMR images, to align all subjects in a common space, to process scar information to obtain physiological volumetric models of scar, and to build 3D models of both the ventricles and the scar regions. A tutorial outlining how to apply the pipeline, which makes use of open-source segmentation and image and mesh processing, is provided. Examples of potential applications of the pipeline to perform electrophysiology simulations or statistical shape modelling in myocardial infarction patients are given. All code is available open-source on Github repository, for use by other researchers.

Acknowledgements. This project was partially funded by the Centre for Cardiological Innovation (CCI), Norway funded by the Norwegian Research Council, and Novo Nordic foundation.

References

1. Arevalo, H.J., Vadakkumpadan, F., Guallar, E., Jebb, A., Malamas, P., Wu, K.C., Trayanova, N.A.: Arrhythmia risk stratification of patients after myocardial infarction using personalized heart models. Nat. Commun. **7** (2016)

---

[14] http://www.cgal.org/.

[15] http://iso2mesh.sourceforge.net/cgi-bin/index.cgi?Home.

[16] https://fenicsproject.org/.

[17] http://www.ecgsim.org.

[18] http://www.cs.ox.ac.uk/chaste/.

[19] https://www.cellml.org/.

[20] http://www.cardiacatlas.org/challenges/lv-statistical-shape-modelling-challenge/.

2. Zhang, X., Cowan, B.R., Bluemke, D.A., Finn, J.P., Fonseca, C.G., Kadish, A.H., Lee, D.C., Lima, J.A., Suinesiaputra, A., Young, A.A., et al.: Atlas-based quantification of cardiac remodeling due to myocardial infarction. PLoS One **9**(10), e110243 (2014)

3. Heiberg, E., Sjgren, J., Ugander, M., Carlsson, M., Engblom, H., Arheden, H.: Design and validation of segment-freely available software for cardiovascular image analysis. BMC Med. Imaging **10**(1) (2010)

4. Heiberg, E., Wigstrom, L., Carlsson, M., Bolger, A., Karlsson, M.: Time resolved three-dimensional automated segmentation of the left ventricle. In: Computers in Cardiology, 2005, pp. 599–602. IEEE (2005)

5. Engblom, H., Tufvesson, J., Jablonowski, R., Carlsson, M., Aletras, A.H., Hoffmann, P., Jacquier, A., Kober, F., Metzler, B., Erlinge, D., et al.: A new automatic algorithm for quantification of myocardial infarction imaged by late gadolinium enhancement cardiovascular magnetic resonance: experimental validation and comparison to expert delineations in multi-center, multi-vendor patient data. J. Cardiovasc. Magn. Reson. **18**(1), 1 (2016)

6. Heiberg, E., Ugander, M., Engblom, H., Gotberg, M., Olivecrona, G.K., Erlinge, D., Arheden, H.: Automated quantification of myocardial infarction from MR images by accounting for partial volume effects: animal, phantom, and human study 1. Radiology **246**(2), 581–588 (2008)

7. Jabbari, R., Engstrøm, T., Glinge, C., Risgaard, B., Jabbari, J., Winkel, B.G., Terkelsen, C.J., Tilsted, H.H., Jensen, L.O., Hougaard, M., et al.: Incidence and risk factors of ventricular fibrillation before primary angioplasty in patients with first st-elevation myocardial infarction: a nationwide study in Denmark. J. Am. Heart Assoc. **4**(1), e001399 (2015)

8. Hergan, K., Schuster, A., Fruhwald, J., Mair, M., Burger, R., Topker, M.: Comparison of left and right ventricular volume measurement using the Simpson's method and the area length method. Eur. J. Radiol. **65**(2), 270–278 (2008)

9. Arevalo, H., Helm, P., Trayanova, N.: Development of a model of the infarcted canine heart that predicts arrhythmia generation from specific cardiac geometry and scar distribution. In: Computers in Cardiology. IEEE 2008, pp. 497–500 (2008)

10. Durrleman, S., Pennec, X., Trouvé, A., Ayache, N.: Statistical models of sets of curves and surfaces based on currents. Med. Image Anal. **13**, 793–808 (2009)

11. Gilbert, K., Lam, H.I., Pontré, B., Cowan, B., Occleshaw, C., Liu, J., Young, A.: An interactive tool for rapid biventricular analysis of congenital heart disease. Clin. Physiol. Funct. Imaging (2015)

12. Pop, M., et al.: EP challenge - STACOM'11: forward approaches to computational electrophysiology using MRI-based models and in-vivo CARTO mapping in swine hearts. In: Camara, O., Konukoglu, E., Pop, M., Rhode, K., Sermesant, M., Young, A. (eds.) STACOM 2011. LNCS, vol. 7085, pp. 1–13. Springer, Heidelberg (2012). doi:10.1007/978-3-642-28326-0_1

Segmentation and Tracking of Myocardial Boundaries Using Dynamic Programming

Athira J. Jacob, Varghese Alex, and Ganapathy Krishnamurthi$^{(\boxtimes)}$

Indian Institute of Technology-Madras, Chennai, India
gankrish@iitm.ac.in

Abstract. Increasing interest in quantification of local myocardial properties throughout the cardiac cycle from tagged MR (tMR) calls for treatment of the cardiac segmentation problem as a spatio-temporal task. The method presented for myocardial segmentation, uses dynamic programming to choose the optimal contour from a set of possible contours subject to maximizing a cost function. Robust Principle Component Analysis (RPCA) is used to decompose the time series into low rank and sparse components and initialization of the contour is done on the low rank approximation. The 3D nature of the images and tag grid location is incorporated into the cost function to get more robust results. 3D+t segmentation of patient data is achieved by propagating contours spatially and temporally. The method is ideal as a pre-processing step in motion quantification and strain rate mapping algorithms.

Keywords: Dynamic programming · Tagged MR image analysis · Robust PCA · Deformable contours · Tracking · 4D cardiac images · Tag

1 Introduction

Currently cardio-vascular magnetic resonance (MR) is the gold standard for assessing global as well as regional heart function due to its high spatial and temporal resolution [2]. In 1988, Zerhouni et al. [9] introduced a MR based noninvasive method for imaging called tagged MRI. Since then tagged MR techniques have shown great potential for noninvasively measuring local mechanical wall function. Segmentation and tracking of the heart wall boundaries and tags is an important step in tMR image analyses tasks. There has been some amount of research efforts on the automated myocardial contour segmentation. Many rely on suppression or removal of tags before segmentation [3,4,8]. Active shape models have been used with learning based methods [6]. Segmentation of tagged MR images still remains a difficult task due to the common presence of cluttered objects, complex object textures, image noise, intensity inhomogeneity, and especially the complexities added by the tagging lines.

We have devised a flexible, fast, non-iterative algorithm that exploits intensity and geometrical priors intrinsic to the image task. It uses Dynamic Programming (DP) to localize the contours and propagate them through subsequent

© Springer International Publishing AG 2017
T. Mansi et al. (Eds.): STACOM 2016, LNCS 10124, pp. 118–126, 2017.
DOI: 10.1007/978-3-319-52718-5_13

spatial and temporal frames. The key contributions of this paper are highlighted as follows

1. Novel use of Stable Principle Components Pursuit (SPCP), a variation of RPCA, to obtain a low rank approximation which is used to automatically obtain initial contour.
2. A robust and effective segmentation framework for segmenting myocardial boundaries in tagged MR images that exploits tag information, which is usually neglected or not well exploited. The method also exploits intensity and geometric information inherent to the images.
3. The spatio-temporal approach of the algorithm makes it suitable to be used along with deformation mapping algorithms of the myocardial tissue.

2   Data

The data used hosted by the Cardiac Atlas Project, originally for the Motion tracking challenge in 2011 [7], consists of 15 scans of healthy volunteers. Each volunteer case consists of cardiac MRI and 3D ultrasound images. The MR acquisition includes: (1) cine SSFP sequences in 2-chamber, 4-chamber, and short-axis views, (2) a whole-heart SSFP sequence gated at end-diastole and end-expiration; and (3) a 4D tMR sequence. The tMR volumes are of size $112 \times 112 \times 111$ (in pixels) with a resolution of $1\,mm/pixel$ and around 25 volumes per cardiac cycle. Tagging is present in three orthogonal directions.

3   Method

Firstly, RPCA and intensity based thresholding is used to initialize a rough endocardium border, which is fit into a circle and sampled to get an initial list of candidate points for endocardium. Using sample points from a circular contour introduces an implicit shape prior and incorporates robustness against missing edges and non-myocardial structures. Each point is used to define a search list around it and DP is used to select one point from each search list by minimizing a cost function. Both geometry and intensity information from the 3D volume is used to define the cost function. The identified endocardial boundary is then used to initialize a rough epicardial boundary and the algorithm proceeds as before except for a change in the cost function. The contours are then propagated spatially and temporally. Apart from traditional applications, this method is particularly suitable for elastography, strain and strain rate imaging etc. to delineate myocardial tissue as the region of interest. The entire procedure of our framework is demonstrated in Fig. 1.

3.1   Robust Principle Component Analyses

Robust PCA (RPCA) [1] is a technique that decomposes a given matrix into a low-rank component and sparse component. In this paper, we have used the

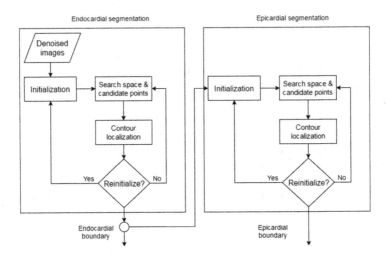

Fig. 1. Workflow of the algorithm

technique of Stable Principle Components Pursuit [10] which seeks an explicit noise component within the RPCA decomposition. If Y is the given matrix of dimensions $N_x N_y \times N_t$, then the method decomposes the matrix into a low-rank matrix L and a sparse matrix S by solving the following convex optimization problem.

$$\min_{L,S} \quad \|L\| + \lambda_{sum}\|S\|_1$$

$$\text{subject to} \quad \|L + S - Y\|_F \leq \epsilon$$

Here $\|.\|_F$ is the Frobenius norm. The 1-norm $\|.\|_1$ and the nuclear norm $\|.\|$ are given by

$$\|S\|_1 = \sum_{(i,j)} \|S_{ij}\|, \|L\| = \sum_i \sigma_i(L)$$

and $\sigma_i(L)$ is the vector of singular values of L.

Physiologically, the low-rank part L appears as a static component while the sparse component S captures motion, in this particular case mostly heartbeats (Fig. 3(b) and (c)). The parameter λ_{sum} controls the relative importance of the low-rank term L vs. the sparse term S, and the parameter ϵ accounts for the unknown perturbations $Y - (L+S)$ in the data not explained by L and S. Higher the λ_{sum} value, faster the convergence rate and sparser the S matrix. The low rank approximation is seen to be robust to the value of λ_{sum}. We have taken $\lambda_{sum} = 0.1$ for the entire study. When $\epsilon = 0$, the SPCP reduces to the standard RPCA problem. ϵ is chosen to be a small value, as 0.05 times the norm of Y.

3.2   Grid Extraction from Tagged MR Images

To deal with 'bleeding' of the contour into the tags, the grid information is incorporated through an additional term in the cost function. The tags in one direction are extracted using a bandpass filter to isolate the spectral peak centered at the lowest harmonic frequency in the corresponding tag direction. The inverse fourier transform of the bandpass region returns a complex harmonic image comprising of a harmonic magnitude image and harmonic phase image. The harmonic phase image gives a detailed picture of the tags. Following edge extraction, a binary image G is obtained from the grid image such that a pixel on the grid and outside the grid gives values of 1 and 0 respectively (Fig. 2).

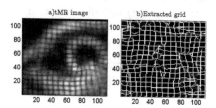

Fig. 2. Raw image (a) and the extracted grid (b)

3.3   Endocardial Segmentation

Initialization. If $N_x \times N_y$ are the dimensions of each image over N_t time points, SPCP is performed on the matrix of dimension $N_x N_y \times N_t$ following intensity homogenization to get a low rank image and sparse component. The low rank image approximates a 'mean' image across all timepoints. The low rank image is pre-processed (Fig. 3(d) and (e)) and an initial boundary is found from this image using intensity based Otsu's method to separate the blood pool from heart walls. The largest non-boundary blob is then extracted to get an initial contour R_{init} for the endocardium.

Contour localization. The initial contour R^{init} is fit to a circle to approximate the ventricle. The circle is then sampled to get M points, $R_1, R_2, R_3 \cdots R_M$, the number of points required in the final contour.

A search space is defined around each point, where it is allowed to move. A point is allowed to move perpendicular to the line joining the previous and next points in the contour. If the mth point of the circular contour is R_m, the search space is defined as from $R_m - q$ to $R_m + q$, in the radial direction, where q is an appropriate search space size (See Fig. 4). To simplify the computation, we choose T points showing highest gradients in the defined direction. Lower T values result in noisier contours whereas higher values result in redundant

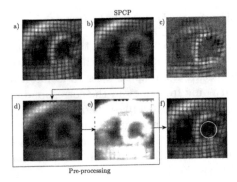

SPCP

Pre-processing

Fig. 3. (a) Original image. (b) Low rank image (c) Sparse image (d) Smoothed Low rank image (e) Histogram truncation (f) Initialized contour fitted into a circle

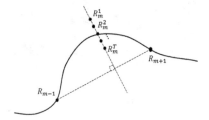

Fig. 4. T candidate points are found around R_{min} the direction perpendicular to the line joining R_{m-1} and R_{m+1}

information with longer computation time. In our case, we have taken $T = 5$ throughout the study.

DP is used to explore the search lists and find the optimal combination based on a cost function, which gives us the final contour R^f.

Cost function: For any endocardial candidate point p with indices (i, j), three terms contribute to the cost associated with that point.

Gradient term: This energy term ensures that the contour is attracted to the edges.

$$F_1 = e^{-\lambda 1 \|\nabla_p I\|} \tag{1}$$

where $\|\nabla_p I\|$ represents the average magnitude of the gradient at point p in image I and its two neighbourhood slices. Using gradient information from three adjacent slices is found to improve robustness and accuracy and is a valid assumption due to thin slices. The grid penalty term described below is used to exclude high gradient terms arising in the tag regions.

Smoothness term: An approximate smoothness term is used,

$$F_2 = e^{-\lambda 2 * \|\|p - C0\| - \|p0 - C0\|\|} \tag{2}$$

where $p0$ is the point preceding the point p in the contour being found and $C0$ is the centre of a circle fitted to initial endocardial boundary R^{init}. This term prevents any drastic changes in relative radii of points and consequently controls the curvature.

Grid penalty: A binary term is used to penalize pixel regions with the tags. The cost of a point p on tagged image with the corresponding grid image G is given by the indicator function

$$F_G = \chi_G(p) \tag{3}$$

F_G is 0 when the point being considered does not fall on any tags. The additional cost from the presence of a tag is $s_G F_G$, where s_G is the corresponding weight. The total cost associated with a point is therefore $s_1 F_1 + s_2 F_2 + s_G F_G$ where s_1, s_2 and s_G are appropriate weights.

3.4   Epicardial Segmentation

Initialization. The delineated endocardial boundary R^f is used in initializing the epicardial boundary. At a point R_m^f on the endocardium, an intensity profile is considered radially and fit to a standard Gaussian. The standard deviation of the Gaussian is taken as the thickness th of the myocardial wall at that point. The corresponding point S_m in the initial epicardial contour is found by displacing R_m^f radially outwards by th to get the initial epicardial contour S^{init}.

Contour localization. S^{init} is fit to a circle and sampled to get N points $S_1, S_2, S_3...S_N$ and search lists of size T are defined around every point. DP is used to explore the search lists and choose points from the candidate points. However a widely observed property of the epicardium is used to make a small modification to the cost function.

Cost function: Epicardial boundaries are often marked by a fall in intensity level, which in addition distinguishes the epicardial boundary from other boundaries nearby. To exploit this information an addition term is used, which we call the falling-edge term.

The falling-edge term at a point p is defined as the difference in directions of the gradient at that point and a ray through p, emanating from the centre. $C0$ is the centre of a circle fitted to initial endocardial boundary R^{init}.

$$F_3 = |\angle \nabla_p I - \angle(C0 - p)| \tag{4}$$

where $\angle$ operator represents the direction. This term is zero when the gradient points to the centre and preferentially supports radially falling gradients. The total cost function for an epicardial point is then, $s_1 F_1 + s_2 F_2 + s_3 F_3 + s_G F_G$, where s_3 is the weight corresponding to F_3. The contours found in one slice are used to propagate both spatially to segment the volume and then temporally to segment all phases of the cardiac cycle.

4   Contour Propagation

The contour initialization is done on an initial slice (mid ventricle) chosen from a volume acquired mid-diastole. Segmentation of the entire volume is done slice by slice. The contour on each slice is initialized using the final contour obtained on the adjacent slice. The final contour of the mid-ventricle slice is then transfered to the mid-ventricle slice of the volume acquired at a successive time point in the cardiac cycle and adjusted using DP (with appropriate cost functions described in the previous sections).

5   Results and Discussion

The algorithm is tested on database of tagged MR cardiac volumes of healthy individuals. Image volumes acquired throughout the cardiac cycle for all patients were segmented. The tMR images are noisy as they capture a single cardiac cycle for all patients. In spite of this, the algorithm gives good contour localization and propagation. Typical segmentation results propagated across the cardiac cycle as well as the volume are shown in Figs. 5 and 6 respectively. Apical slices give slightly less accurate segmentation results due to their difficulty in segmentation. The results are almost instantaneous due to the computational simplicity.

Propagating the contours sometimes result in the contours accumulating errors due to weak boundaries, noise, sudden geometry changes etc. This can be remedied by re-initialization of the contour. The algorithm also faces difficulty in providing accurate results at the apical slices. The cost function is

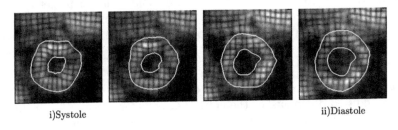

i)Systole   ii)Diastole

Fig. 5. Results of segmentation propagated across time

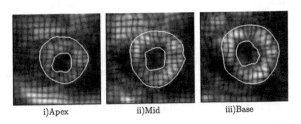

i)Apex   ii)Mid   iii)Base

Fig. 6. Segmentation propagated across volume. Slices at apical, mid and basal level are shown

Table 1. Hyper-parameters used

	Endocardium			Epicardium			
Parameters	$\lambda 1, s_1$	$\lambda 2, s_2$	s_G	$\lambda 1, s_1$	$\lambda 2, s_2$	s_3	s_G
Values	3,3	0.1,1.2	0.45	3,3	0.1,0.3	0.2	0.4

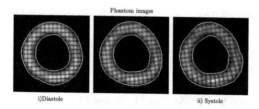

Fig. 7. Validation on cardiac phantom

tuned by setting $\lambda 1$ and s_1 to adjust the gradient term. For epicardium, the falling-edge term is increased to around a third of the gradient term. Then the smoothing term is increased to smooth out kinks in the curve while maintaining the shape. The grid penalty term, if present, is adjusted to a similar range as that of smoothing term. The values of the various hyper-parameters used for segmenting patient volumes are given in Table 1. The hyper-parametes are tuned on one patient and the algorithm performs effectively on the other volumes. It is expected that for images acquired using different scanners the parameters would have to be modified and validated using representative data-sets.

Unlike methods that require specific shape templates for points in the cardiac cycle, using image cues and gradients, the proposed method is able to segment the myocardium (and the LV) over all cardiac phases. This makes the algorithm suitable for region of interest analysis of displacement fields in the myocardium. Our method uses the tag grids to modify the cost function and has minimal computational cost since the tag extraction is done in most algorithms to calculate displacement fields and strain rates [5]. We validated our method qualitatively on the cardiac phantom which mimics the cardiac cycle (Fig. 7). The inner and outer walls are localized accurately which is evident on visual inspection. Our method as presented, would be an excellent pre-processing tool for cardiac deformation analysis algorithms. Since methods like HARP contain grid extraction as a necessary step, the computational demand is also lower. The validation done here ascertains that the myocardium is isolated from the background tissue effectively. For applications that involve estimating LVEF, systolic and diastolic volumes, a thorough validation in the form of dice scores or Hausdorff distance against expert drawn contours would be required.

6   Conclusion

In this paper, we have presented a method to extract the contours of the myocardium in tagged MR cardiac volumes. Contour initialization is done using SPCP and propagated by minimizing(using DP) a cost function based on inherent image properties. It is able to successfully segment tagged MR images which pose serious challenges to traditional methods due to the presence of tags. The method is particularly suitable as a pre-processing step for cardiac deformation analysis & strain rate imaging.

References

1. Candès, E.J., Li, X., Ma, Y., Wright, J.: Robust principal component analysis? J. ACM (JACM) **58**(3), 11 (2011)
2. Edvardsen, T., Gerber, B.L., Garot, J., Bluemke, D.A., Lima, J.A., Smiseth, O.A.: Quantitative assessment of intrinsic regional myocardial deformation by doppler strain rate echocardiography in humans: validation against three-dimensional tagged magnetic resonance imaging. Circulation **106**(1), 50–56 (2002). doi:10.1161/01.CIR.0000019907.77526.75. http://circ.ahajournals.org/content/106/1/50.abstract
3. Guttman, M., Prince, J., McVeigh, E.: Tag and contour detection in tagged MR images of the left ventricle. IEEE Trans. Med. Imaging **13**(1), 74–88 (1994). doi:10.1109/42.276146. ISSN 0278-0062
4. Metaxas, D.N., Axel, L., Qian, Z., Huang, X.: A segmentation and tracking system for 4D cardiac tagged MR images, pp. 1541–1544 (2006)
5. Osman, N.F., Kerwin, W.S., McVeigh, E.R., Prince, J.L.: Cardiac motion tracking using CINE harmonic phase (HARP) magnetic resonance imaging. Magn. Reson. Med. Official J. Soc. Magn. Reson. Med./Soc. Magn. Reson. Med. **42**(6), 1048 (1999)
6. Qian, Z., Metaxas, D.N., Axel, L.: A learning framework for the automatic and accurate segmentation of cardiac tagged MRI images. In: Liu, Y., Jiang, T., Zhang, C. (eds.) CVBIA 2005. LNCS, vol. 3765, pp. 93–102. Springer, Heidelberg (2005). doi:10.1007/11569541_11
7. Tobon-Gomez, C., De Craene, M., Mcleod, K., Tautz, L., Shi, W., Hennemuth, A., Prakosa, A., Wang, H., Carr-White, G., Kapetanakis, S., et al.: Benchmarking framework for myocardial tracking and deformation algorithms: an open access database. Med. Image Anal. **17**(6), 632–648 (2013)
8. Yang, X., Murase, K.: Tagged cardiac MR image segmentation by contrast enhancement and texture analysis, pp. 4–210 (2009)
9. Zerhouni, E.A., Parish, D.M., Rogers, W.J., Yang, A., Shapiro, E.P.: Human heart: tagging with MR imaging-a method for noninvasive assessment of myocardial motion. Radiology **169**(1), 59–63 (1988). doi:10.1148/radiology.169.1.3420283. http://dx.doi.org/10.1148/radiology.169.1.3420283
10. Zhou, Z., Li, X., Wright, J., Candes, E., Ma, Y.: Stable principal component pursuit. In: IEEE International Symposium on Information Theory Proceedings (ISIT), pp. 1518–1522. IEEE (2010)

Registration with Adjacent Anatomical Structures for Cardiac Resynchronization Therapy Guidance

Daniel Toth[1,2]($\boxtimes$), Maria Panayiotou[2], Alexander Brost[3],
Jonathan M. Behar[2,4], Christopher A. Rinaldi[2,4], Kawal S. Rhode[2],
and Peter Mountney[5]

[1] Siemens Healthcare Ltd., Camberley, UK
daniel.toth@kcl.ac.uk
[2] Division of Imaging Sciences and Biomedical Engineering,
King's College London, London, England, UK
[3] Siemens Healthcare GmbH, Erlangen, Germany
[4] Department of Cardiology,
Guy's and St. Thomas' Hospitals NHS Foundation Trust, London, UK
[5] Medical Imaging Technologies, Siemens Healthcare, Princeton, NJ, USA

Abstract. The clinical applications and benefits of multi-modal image registration are wide-ranging and well established. Current image based approaches exploit cross-modality information, such as landmarks or anatomical structures, which is visible in both modalities. A lack of cross-modality information can prohibit accurate automatic registration. This paper proposes a novel approach for MR to X-ray image registration which uses prior knowledge of adjacent anatomical structures to enable registration without cross-modality image information. The registration of adjacent structures formulated as a partial surface registration problem which is solved using a globally optimal ICP method. The practical clinical application of the approach is demonstrated on an image guided cardiac resynchronization therapy procedure. The left ventricle (segmented from pre-operative MR) is registered to the coronary vessel tree (extracted from intra-operative fluoroscopic images). The proposed approach is validated on synthetic and phantom data, where the results show a good comparison with the ground truth registrations. The vertex-to-vertex MAE was 3.28 ± 1.18 mm for 10 X-ray image pairs of the phantom.

1 Introduction

Multi-modal image registration is a fundamental research area in medical imaging. Spatially aligning complementary information from two or more imaging modalities has a wide range of applications, including diagnostics, planning, simulation and guidance.

Registration of multiple modalities has been extensively studied and many solutions have been proposed [1] using landmarks, image intensity, gradients,

© Springer International Publishing AG 2017
T. Mansi et al. (Eds.): STACOM 2016, LNCS 10124, pp. 127–134, 2017.
DOI: 10.1007/978-3-319-52718-5_14

mutual information and learning similarity functions. These approaches often assume cross-modality information, e.g., anatomical structures, landmarks or objects that are visible in both imaging modalities. The presence of cross-modality information is a reasonable assumption for many clinical applications. However, the lack of such information can prohibit automatic and accurate registration.

In image guided interventions, such as cardiac resynchronization therapy (CRT), pre-operative MR or SPECT images are used to analyse tissue characteristics or function and intraoperative X-ray fluoroscopy is used to guide the procedure. The pre- and intra-operative modalities are fundamentally different and do not share significant cross-modality information. In such cases alternative registration strategies are required.

Cross-modality registration for CRT procedures can be performed using fiducial markers and optical tracking devices [2], however, this requires the pre-operative MR imaging immediately before the procedure and additional hardware in the operating room. Anatomical registration has been proposed where the position of the vessels is inferred from catheters and aligned to vessels segmented from pre-operative images [3,4]. However, catheters may induce deformations in the anatomy and the quality of MR images may be too low to identify vascular structures accurately. Registration of pre-operative SPECT to fluoroscopic images has been proposed by manually matching landmarks (intraventricular grooves to coronary artery tree), performing an iterative closest point (ICP) refinement and finally a non linear warping [5]. This method is dependent on accurately identifying landmarks in pre-operative data which is challenging and variations of the anatomy may result in inaccuracies. Additionally, since the epicardium is not visible in the SPECT images, the center of the myocardium is detected and a constant myocardial thickness is assumed. Considering this, and that the vessels are warped to the generated epicardial surface, the accuracy of the algorithm is questionable.

In this paper, a novel approach is presented for registering multi-modal images by using adjacent anatomical structures which does not rely on cross-modality information. The registration of adjacent structures is formulated as a partial surface registration problem which is solved using a globally optimal ICP (Go-ICP) algorithm. The practical clinical application is demonstrated on an image guided CRT procedure by registering the left ventricle (LV) (pre-operative MR) to the coronary vessel anatomy (intra-operative fluoroscopy). The method is validated on synthetic and phantom data.

2   Methods

At the core of the proposed registration approach is the use of anatomical structures that are adjacent or share a common surface. For example, in cardiac anatomy the epicardial surface of the LV is adjacent to the coronary sinus (CS) vessel tree. The LV is visible in preoperative MR but the vessel tree is not. The vessel tree is visible during contrast injected X-ray fluoroscopy, however, the LV is not. This concept is illustrated in Fig. 1. The following section outlines how this prior anatomical knowledge can be exploited to register multi-modal images without cross-modality image information.

2.1 Extracting Adjacent Anatomical Structures

The LV is automatically segmented from pre-operative MRI. The epicardial contour is detected in long (two-, three- and four-chamber) and short axis images using a combination of machine learning landmark detection and gray level analysis [6]. A mesh is fit to the contours to generate a surface representation of the LV epicardium at end diastole as shown in Fig. 1(a).

Two contrast injected fluoroscopy images are acquired during the intervention. The images and the corresponding venous tree (CS and the venous branches that drain into the CS) are illustrated in Fig. 1(b). The sequences are acquired at different angulations and time points. As a result the sequences capture the anatomy at various points in the cardiac cycle. One (end diastolic) frame from each sequence is automatically selected using masked principle component analysis motion gating [7]. In the method, cardiac motion is extracted by band pass filtering the variation of the first principle component. Corresponding points on the CS are manually selected and reconstructed by epipolar triangulation to create a point cloud that represents the venous tree in 3D.

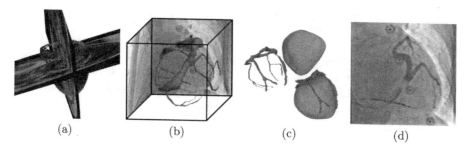

(a)   (b)   (c)   (d)

Fig. 1. Registration of adjacent landmarks in a cardiac procedure. (a) The MR data is segmented to extract the LV epicardial mesh (green). (b) The point cloud of the coronary vasculature (red) is reconstructed from two contrast injected venograms. (c) The segmented LV mesh is registered to the reconstructed point cloud (d) to show a valid overlay that can be used for interventional guidance. (Color figure online)

2.2 Registration Algorithm

Registering the reconstructed vessel point cloud x (data) and the vertices of the LV epicardial shell y (model) can be described as a partial point cloud matching problem with unknown point correspondences and can be formulated as

$$E(\boldsymbol{R},\boldsymbol{t}) = \sum_{i=1}^{N} e_i^2(\boldsymbol{R},\boldsymbol{t}) = \sum_{i=1}^{N} ||\boldsymbol{R}\boldsymbol{x}_i + \boldsymbol{t} - \boldsymbol{y}_{j*}||^2, \tag{1}$$

where e_i is the error of point i depending on the rotation $\mathbf{R}$ and the translation t, N represents the number of data points and $\mathbf{y}_{j*}$ the optimal correspondences. However, j^* is a function of $\mathbf{R}$, t and $\mathbf{x}_i$. If the optimal $\mathbf{R}$ and t were known, the correspondences could be found easily and if the correspondences were known, the optimal $\mathbf{R}$ and t would be easy to calculate. The well established approach for such a problem is the ICP algorithm, however, it always finds the nearest local minimum. To find the global minimum, the Branch and Bound (BnB) algorithm can be used [8]. Convergence to the optimal solution is guaranteed, however, the whole search space may have to be processed.

BnB and ICP were combined to overcome their individual weaknesses, thus to provide a fast globally optimal solution [9]. The search space for the registrations is the special Euclidean group $SE(3)$, that incorporates all real 3D motions and can be subdivided into the rotation group $SO(3)$ and the translations of $\mathbb{R}^3$. $SO(3)$ is parametrized by a solid sphere of radius π, and is simplified by using the cube $[-\pi, \pi]^3$. The translations in $\mathbb{R}^3$ can be parametrized by a cube $[-\xi, \xi]^3$, where ξ is the half side length of the cube.

The algorithm uses two priority lists, one for the rotation cubes C_r in the outer BnB, and one for the translation cubes C_t in the inner BnB. The lower the lower error bound of a cube, the higher its priority in the list. The outer BnB calculates the lower bound

$$E \doteq \sum_{i=1}^N e_i^2 = \sum_{i=1}^N \max(e_i(\mathbf{R}_{r_0}, t_0) - \gamma, 0)^2 \tag{2}$$

for the initial cube, where (r_0, t_0) represents the center of the 3D motion domain $C_r \times C_t$ and γ is the uncertainty radius [10]. If the current error estimate E^* is close to E, the solution is found. Otherwise, the cube is subdivided and the subcubes are processed. The upper error bound

$$\overline{E} \doteq \sum_{i=1}^N \overline{e}_i^2 = \sum_{i=1}^N e_i^2(\mathbf{R}_{r_0}, t_0), \tag{3}$$

and the corresponding optimal translation is calculated for each subcube C_t by the inner BnB algorithm. If the upper error bound is smaller than E^*, ICP is run to update the error and the transformation $(\mathbf{R}, t)$. The lower error bound $\underline{E}$ for the current subcube is calculated and if it is above E^*, the cube is discarded, otherwise it is added to the priority list. The above steps, starting with removing the first item from the priority list are repeated until the lower error bound and the current error estimate are both within a set threshold $(\underline{E} - E^* < \text{tresh})$.

The algorithm guarantees convergence to the globally optimal solution. It is additionally much more efficient than the standard BnB algorithm, since even if it explores the whole possible solution space, it refines the intermediate results with the ICP method, thus benefitting from the good attributes of both algorithms. It has been shown that the algorithm is well suited to registering partial surfaces, has high noise tolerance and is robust to outliers [10].

3   Results and Evaluation

The evaluation of the approach on *in vivo* patient data is extremely challenging. The lack of cross-modality information in the available images makes the generation of an accurate ground truth registration very difficult, since no automatic approach is capable of registering the images and there is only minimal information present (heart shadow) for a clinical expert to perform the registration manually. Therefore, the proposed method was quantitatively and qualitatively evaluated on synthetic and phantom data. The practical clinical application is demonstrated on a CRT intervention.

3.1   Synthetic Data

A synthetic dataset of the LV and coronary tree was created from a patient MR dataset. The LV point cloud is segmented from MR as described above, however, the coronary tree is not visible in the MR and therefore it is artificially created by sampling points from the vertices of the LV mesh. Four experiments were performed to evaluate the proposed approach.

A baseline comparison between ICP and Go-ICP was performed by registering two LV meshes to each other where one mesh was artificially transformed by a rotation (-25° to 25° around all three axis with 5° steps). For each initialization the mean absolute error (MAE) of the corresponding vertices (vertex-to-vertex error) was calculated, see Table 1. The Go-ICP method always finds the optimal alignment, compared to the high fail rate (MAE > 5.0mm) of the conventional ICP method. The registration of the coronary tree to the LV is a partial registration problem. An experiment was performed to determine the minimum number of coronary tree points required for a successful registration, the datapoints were a random subset of the model vertices and the number of the randomly selected vertices was varied. The average error decreases significantly as the number of selected points increases. A minimum of 20 points representing the coronary tree was chosen since then the error decreases below 0.025 mm.

Partial surface registration performance was evaluated with ICP and Go-ICP using 20 points to represent the coronary tree and transforming the data as described above. The results shown in Table 1 demonstrate the proposed approach is robust even in the partial surface registration. To inspect the noise

Table 1. Results of the evaluation performed on the synthetic data for registering the complete mesh and only a subset of the vertices (point cloud) with the ICP and the Go-ICP methods.

	Mesh		Pt. cloud	
	ICP	Go-ICP	ICP	Go-ICP
Mean MAE (mm)	12.59	0.00	18.76	0.02
Std. dev. (mm)	3.92	0.00	6.92	0.03
Fail rate (%)	99.10	0.00	98.90	0.00

tolerance of the method the same, 20 vertex, realistic point cloud was used as in the previous experiment. In addition to the transformation, white Gaussian noise was added to the data with varying standard deviation. For no added noise the vertex-to-vertex error is close to 0, however, as the noise increases from 1 mm to 2 mm, the error increases from 1.63 ± 0.12 mm to 3.68 ± 2.02 mm.

3.2 Phantom Data

Phantom experiments were performed to evaluate the proposed approach in a clinical imaging environment with known ground truth. The LV epicardial surface (segmented from an MR) was 3D printed and wires were attached to model the vascular tree. Intra-operative ground truth data was obtained by acquiring a cone beam CT (CBCT). The LV point cloud, from CBCT, was registered to ten pairs of X-ray fluoroscopy.

The mean 3D vertex-to-vertex MAE between the ground truth and the automatically registered mesh was 3.28 ± 1.18 mm. The mean Hausdorff (surface-to-surface) distance was 1.12 mm with a mean maximal distance of 3.36 mm. The mean Dice score of the projections was 0.98 ± 0.01. A summary of the results can be seen in Table 2. The overlay and the Hausdorff distance mapping is shown for one setup in Fig. 2. Small registration errors are attributed to inaccuracies in the reconstruction of the vascular tree and LV segmentation.

3.3 Clinical Application

The practical clinical application of the approach is demonstrated on a CRT procedure, see Fig. 3. The clinician must place electrodes in healthy tissue, however, it is not possible to differentiate between healthy and scarred tissue using conventional X-ray fluoroscopy guidance. Scar tissue (red), segmented from late gadolinium enhancement MR images, can be overlaid onto X-ray fluoroscopy images using the proposed approach, after the acquisition of two contrasted venograms. The presented overlay of scar tissue meshes onto X-ray fluoroscopy guides the clinician towards healthy tissue which can potentially increase responder rates and reduce procedure time. Since the orientation of the heart is approximately known, the rotation space was limited to $\pm 25°$ in all three degrees of freedom. The registration time with the set limits for the case was 45 s on an Intel i7 with 8 GB of RAM.

Table 2. Quantitative results of the evaluation on phantom data. The vertex-to-vertex MAE was calculated in 2D and 3D, the dice score in 2D and the Hausdorff distance in 3D for the ground truth and the automatically registered meshes.

	2D	3D
MAE (mm)	2.79 ± 0.68	3.28 ± 1.18
Dice score	0.98 ± 0.01	
Hausdorff distance (mm)		1.12 (max. 3.36)

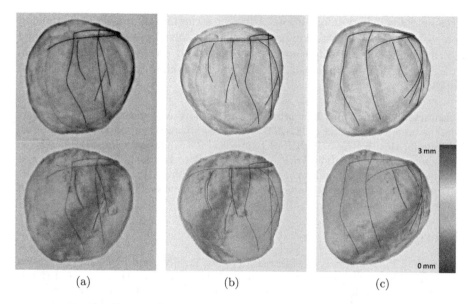

Fig. 2. (a) Anterior-posterior (AP 0°), (b) right anterior oblique (RAO 30°) and (c) left anterior oblique (LAO 30°) X-ray projections of the LV Phantom with the Hausdorff distance mapped to the surface vertex color. (Color figure online)

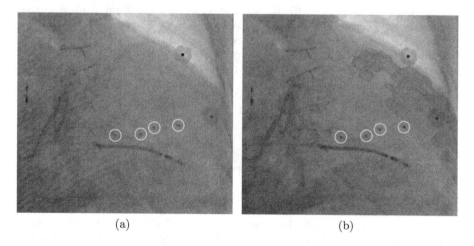

Fig. 3. Registration application for a CRT procedure. (a) Overlay of the epicardal mesh (green) and (b) the segmented scar tissue mesh (red). The electrodes of the multipolar lead (yellow) are placed to avoid scar tissue. (Color figure online)

4   Conclusion

This paper presents a novel method for automated registration of multi-modal images using adjacent anatomical structures. The approach does not use cross-modality image information. Adjacent structure alignment is formulated as a partial surface registration problem which is solved using a globally optimal ICP method. The presented approach is validated on synthetic and phantom data. The method is capable of fast registration making it well suited to clinical workflows.

Acknowledgements and Disclaimer. The authors are grateful for the support from the Innovate UK grant 32684-234174. The research was supported by the National Institute for Health Research (NIHR) Biomedical Research Centre based at Guys and St Thomas NHS Foundation Trust and Kings College London. The views expressed are those of the authors and not necessarily those of the NHS, NIHR or the Department of Health. Concepts and information presented are based on research and are not commercially available.

References

1. Markelj, P., Tomaževič, D., Likar, B., Pernuš, F.: A review of 3D/2D registration methods for image-guided interventions. Med. Image Anal. **16**(3), 642–661 (2012)
2. Rhode, K.S., Hill, D.L.G., Edwards, P.J., Hipwell, J., Rueckert, D., Sanchez-Ortiz, G., Hegde, S., Rahunathan, V., Razavi, R.: Registration and tracking to integrate X-ray and MR images in an XMR facility. IEEE Trans. Med. Imaging **22**(11), 1369–1378 (2003)
3. Truong, M.V.N., Aslam, A., Rinaldi, C.A., Razavi, R., Penney, G.P., Rhode, K.: Preliminary investigation: 2D–3D registration of MR and X-ray cardiac images using catheter constraints. In: MICCAI Workshop on Cardiovascular Interventional Imaging and Biophysical Modelling, London, pp. 1–9 (2009)
4. Bourier, F., Brost, A., Yatziv, L., Hornegger, J., Strobel, N., Kurzidim, K.: Coronary sinus extraction for multimodality registration to guide transseptal puncture. In: 8th Interventional MRI Symposium, Leipzig, pp. 311–313 (2010)
5. Faber, T.L., Santana, C.A., Garcia, E.V., Candell-Riera, J., Folks, R.D., Peifer, J.W., Hopper, A., Aguade, S., Angel, J., Klein, J.L.: Three-dimensional fusion of coronary arteries with myocardial perfusion distributions: clinical validation. J. Nuclear Med. **45**(5), 745–753 (2004)
6. Jolly, M.-P., Guetter, C., Lu, X., Xue, H., Guehring, J.: Automatic segmentation of the myocardium in cine MR images using deformable registration. In: Camara, O., Konukoglu, E., Pop, M., Rhode, K., Sermesant, M., Young, A. (eds.) STACOM 2011. LNCS, vol. 7085, pp. 98–108. Springer, Heidelberg (2012). doi:10.1007/978-3-642-28326-0_10
7. Panayiotou, M., King, A.P., Housden, R.J., Ma, Y., Cooklin, M., O'Neill, M., Gill, J., Rinaldi, C.A., Rhode, K.S.: A statistical method for retrospective cardiac and respiratory motion gating of interventional cardiac x-ray images. Med. Phys. **41**(7), 071901 (2014)
8. Dakin, R.J.: A tree-search algorithm for mixed integer programming problems. Comput. J. **8**(3), 250–255 (1965)
9. Yang, J., Li, H., Jia, Y.: Go-ICP: solving 3D registration efficiently and globally optimally. In: 2013 IEEE International Conference on Computer Vision, pp. 1457–1464 (2013)
10. Yang, J., Li, H., Campbell, D., Jia, Y.: Go-ICP: a globally optimal solution to 3D ICP point-set registration. IEEE Trans. Pattern Anal. Mach. Intell. **PP**(99), 1–14 (2015)

Estimation of Purkinje Activation from ECG: An Intermittent Left Bundle Branch Block Study

Sophie Giffard-Roisin[1](✉), Lauren Fovargue[2], Jessica Webb[2], Roch Molléro[1], Jack Lee[2], Hervé Delingette[1], Nicholas Ayache[1], Reza Razavi[2], and Maxime Sermesant[1]

[1] Inria, Asclepios Research Project, Sophia Antipolis, France
sophie.giffard-roisin@inria.fr
[2] Department of Biomedical Engineering, King's College London, London, UK

Abstract. Modelling the cardiac electrophysiology (EP) can help understand pathologies and predict the response to therapies such as cardiac resynchronization. To this end, estimating patient-specific model parameters is crucial. In the case of patients with bundle branch blocks (BBB), part of the Purkinje system is often affected. The aim of this work is to estimate the activation of the right and left Purkinje systems from standard non-invasive techniques: magnetic resonance imaging (MRI) and 12-lead electrocardiogram (ECG). As it is difficult to differentiate the contribution of the Purkinje system, this work relies on a particular intermittent left BBB (LBBB) case where both LBBB and absence of LBBB (ALBBB) were recorded on different 12-lead ECGs. First, an efficient forward EP model is proposed by coupling a Mitchell-Schaeffer cardiac model with a current dipole formulation that simulates the ECG. We used the Covariance Matrix Adaptation Evolution Strategy (CMA-ES) algorithm to optimize the 3 parameters by minimizing the error with the real ECG. The estimation of conduction velocity (CV) parameters for LBBB and ALBBB shows a good agreement on the myocardial CV ($0.39\,\mathrm{m/s}$ for ABBB, $0.40\,\mathrm{m/s}$ for LBBB), while the estimation of the left Purkinje CV seems to identify the pathology ($1.32\,\mathrm{m/s}$ for ALBBB, $0.49\,\mathrm{m/s}$ for LBBB). Finally, the plots of the simulated 12-lead ECGs together with the ground truth ECGs indicate similar shapes.

Keywords: Electrophysiology · Electrophysiological model · Forward EP model · Parameter estimation · Purkinje system

1 Introduction

Modelling the cardiac electrophysiology (EP) can help understanding pathologies and predicting the response to therapies such as cardiac resynchronization therapies (CRT). To this end, estimating patient-specific model parameters is

© Springer International Publishing AG 2017
T. Mansi et al. (Eds.): STACOM 2016, LNCS 10124, pp. 135–142, 2017.
DOI: 10.1007/978-3-319-52718-5_15

crucial. In the case of patients with bundle branch blocks (BBB), part of the Purkinje system is often affected. The Purkinje fibers are located just beneath the endocardium and are able to conduct cardiac action potentials quickly and efficiently: typical conduction velocity (CV) ranges from 2 to 3 m/s while it ranges from 0.3 to 0.4 m/s for myocardial cells [1]. Stimulus arrives from the atrioventricular node through the His bundle and separate the network in two branches, the left bundle and the right bundle. When a block occurs in a bundle (LBBB for left, RBBB for right), the Purkinje system is not as efficient and the contraction of the ventricles isn't synchronized.

Some studies have been focusing on the understanding of LBBB patterns by simulating ECGs with different parameters from precise cardiac and torso models [2,3]. Because of their complexity, we defined a simpler model for the estimation of patient-specific parameters. A study has also recently proposed an EP parameter estimation from ECG data [4]. It uses two features from the 12-lead ECG to recover 3 electrical diffusivity parameters using a boundary element method forward model and a polynomial regression. As it is difficult to differentiate the contribution of the Purkinje system, our work relies on a particular intermittent LBBB case where both LBBB and absence of LBBB (ALBBB) are recorded on 12-lead ECGs. First, an efficient forward EP model is proposed by coupling a 3-parameter cardiac EP model based on the Mitchell-Schaeffer model with a current dipole formulation. We used the CMA-ES algorithm to optimize the 3 parameters by minimizing the error with the ECG signals.

2   Materials and Methods

2.1   Clinical Data

In this study, we considered cardiac imaging data from MRI and electrical data from the 12-lead ECG. The MRI acquisition allows a precise myocardial geometry at end diastole. The 12-lead ECG represents the cardiac electrical activity recorded from 9 body surface electrodes. Because the locations of the electrodes were not registered, we manually position them guided by the conventional ECG placement (Fig. 1(a)). The 12 standard Einthoven, Goldberger and Wilson leads (12-lead ECG) measures the potential differences between selected electrodes.

2.2   Pre-processing

The myocardial mesh was generated using the VP2HF platform [6] and the VP2HF meshing pipeline[1] creating a tetrahedral mesh with roughly 90 K tetrahedra. Rule-based fibre directions were estimated with an elevation angle between −70° and 70°. The right and left Purkinje regions were manually delineated (Fig. 1(b)). The 12-lead ECG were digitized using the opensource Engauge Digitizer followed by a resampling at a rate of 1 kHz. Only the 200 ms following the Q wave were used (QRS window).

---

[1] VP2HF is a European Seventh Framework Program, http://www.vp2hf.eu/. The VP2HF meshing pipeline is based on CGAL, VTK, ITK and VMTK opensources libraries.

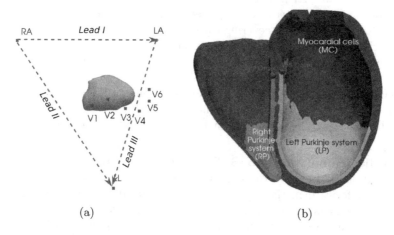

(a) (b)

Fig. 1. (a) The 9 ECG electrodes and the cardiac mesh. (b) Long axis view of the cardiac mesh with delineated regions: Myocardial cells region (blue), right Purkinje system region (orange) and left Purkinje system region (beige). The red dots are the modeled right and left onset activation locations (Color figure online).

2.3 Forward EP Model

Mitchell-Schaeffer Cardiac Model: We simulated the electrical activation of the heart using the monodomain version of the Mitchell-Schaeffer's EP model [7]. The monodomain formulation considers that the extra-cellular and intra-cellular anisotropies are proportional and therefore we can solve directly the transmembrane potential. It is governed by:

$$C_m \frac{\partial v}{\partial t} + I_{ion} = \nabla \cdot \boldsymbol{\sigma} \nabla v \qquad (1)$$

with v the transmembrane potential, C_m the membrane capacitance and I_{ion} the current through the cell membrane per unit of area. The anisotropic conduction tensor $\boldsymbol{\sigma}$ is defined as $\boldsymbol{\sigma} = \sigma \cdot diag(1, r, r)$ where the anisotropy ratio r enables conduction velocity in the fibre direction to be larger than in the transverse plane (we used $r = (1/2.5)^2$). The conductivity σ is a local parameter that depends on the capability of the tissue to propagate the electrical activation. σ can be written in terms of intracellular and extracellular conductivities: $\sigma = \frac{\sigma^i \sigma^e}{\sigma^i + \sigma^e}$. The reduction of the monodomain model implies $\sigma^i = \lambda \sigma^e$ for some scalar λ resulting in a linear relationship between σ and σ^i. The diffusivity d (in $m^2 s^{-1}$) can be expressed as a conductivity σ (in $\Omega.m$) by using $\sigma = C_m \beta\, d$ with C_m the membrane capacitance and β the surface-to-volume ratio. Finally, the diffusion d is linked to the conduction velocity c in m/s by $c = k\sqrt{d}$, where the constant k was estimated numerically in our simulations as $0.35\,s^{-1/2}$.

In this work, we considered 3 different domains with uniform conduction velocities: the myocardial cells (MC), the left Purkinje system (LP) and the right Purkinje system (RP). The MC was modelled as one single domain for simplification reasons and because the patient was non-ischaemic. We modelled the LP and RP as a thin layer covering the endocardial surfaces. By considering that the Purkinje geometry is unknown, this simplification to a layer allows also a rapid computation. Concretely, the layer is composed of all the tetrahedra connected to the endocardial surface.

We manually selected the onset activation locations on the septum near the valves, see Fig. 1(b). This was driven by the fact that the electrical wave arrives from the His bundle to the left and right bundles located on the septum.

From Cardiac Simulations to BSPM, Current Dipole Formulation: We computed simultaneously the cardiac electrical sources and body surface potentials. Our forward method is based on a simplified framework composed of sources and sensors in an infinite and homogeneous domain. As in [5], we modelled every myocardium volume element (tetrahedron) as a spatially fixed but time varying current dipole. The equivalent current density $\mathbf{j}_{eq}$ writes as:

$$\mathbf{j}_{eq} = -\sigma^i \nabla v \qquad (2)$$

$\mathbf{j}_{eq}$ is a current dipole moment per unit of volume and the local dipole moment $\mathbf{p}$ in the volume V writes as $\mathbf{p} = \int_V \mathbf{j}_{eq} dV$. According to the volume conductor theory, the electric potential at a distance R in a homogeneous volume conductor of conductivity σ_T is:

$$\Psi(R) = \frac{1}{4\pi\sigma_T} \int_V \mathbf{j}_{eq} \cdot \nabla(\frac{1}{R}) dV \qquad (3)$$

The infinitesimal dipole moment of the volume dV_X located at position X is defined as $\mathbf{p}_X = \mathbf{j}_{eq,X} \, dV_X = -\sigma_X^i \nabla v_X dV_X$. As we use linear tetrahedra in the FEM discretization of the myocardium, the potential v is linear and ∇v is constant over the tetrahedron. We get the following formulation of the dipole moment of the charge in the volume V_H of tetrahedron H of the myocardial mesh: $\mathbf{p}_H = -\sigma_H^i \nabla v_H V_H$. From [8], the gradient of the electric potential in tetrahedron H can be computed from the potentials $v(X_H^k)$ at the nodes X_H^k, and the contribution Ψ_H of the tetrahedron H to the potential field calculated at position X_T is:

$$\Psi_H(X_T) = \frac{1}{4\pi\sigma_T} \frac{\sigma_H^i V_H (\nabla v_H \cdot \overrightarrow{HT})}{\|\overrightarrow{HT}\|^3} \qquad (4)$$

with $\overrightarrow{HT}$ the vector from centre of the tetrahedron H to the torso electrode location T. Finally, we sum over the whole mesh to get the potential field at X_T. The implementation was performed using the SOFA platform[2], with a direct coupling to the Mitchell-Schaeffer model. One iteration of the model is computed in 0.1 ms (dual-Xeon X6570 with 12 cores at 2.93 GHz).

---

[2] SOFA is an Open Source medical simulation software available at http://www. sofa-framework.org.

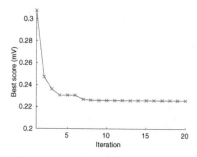

Fig. 2. Best score versus the number of iterations of the CMA-ES algorithm. The score is identified as the mean error between the simulated and real 12-lead ECG, in mV.

2.4 Parameter Estimation Using CMA-ES Algorithm

We estimated the 3 conduction parameters using a Covariance Matrix Adaptation Evolution Strategy (CMA-ES) [9]. It is a derivative-free and stochastic algorithm that is suited for non-convex continuous optimization problems. At each iteration, new candidate solutions are sampled from a multivariate normal distribution whose covariance matrix is adapted according to the ranking between the candidate solutions of the previous iteration. We define the score of a simulation S as its error to the ground truth 12-lead ECGs Ψ_{GT}:

$$f(S) = \int_{t=0}^{T} \frac{1}{N} \sum_{i=1}^{N} |\Psi_{GT}(i,t) - \frac{\|\Psi_{GT}\|}{\|\Psi_S\|} \Psi_S(i,t)| \tag{5}$$

with N the number of leads ($N = 12$), T the final time (T = 200 ms), $\Psi_{GT}(i,t)$ the ground truth difference of potential of the lead i at time t and $\Psi_S(i,t)$ the simulated difference of potential of the lead i at time t. We used a population of 100 simulations per generation and optimized over 20 generations. We initialized the algorithm by a multivariate distribution of mean $x_0 = (0.6,0.6,0.6)$ m/s and standard deviation std = 0.1 m/s in each direction. We fix the parameter searching range at $[0.05, 2.5]$ m/s to avoid non-physical solutions. The best score vs, the number of iterations for a parameter estimation is plotted on Fig. 2.

Table 1. Estimated conduction velocities for LBBB and ALBBB.

CV (m/s)	Myocardium	Left Purkinje	Right Purkinje
Initially	0.6	0.6	0.6
LBBB	0.39	0.49	0.95
Absence of LBBB	0.40	1.32	1.22

3   Evaluation on an Intermittent LBBB Patient

3.1   Intermittent LBBB Patient Data

As an evaluation of the proposed method, a patient with intermittent LBBB was chosen. The data has been acquired at St Thomas Hospital (London) as part of the VP2HF project. Both LBBB pattern and absence of LBBB (ALBBB) were documented on two 12-lead ECG, the ALBBB being recorded after the LBBB. The parameters were estimated separately for the LBBB and ALBBB. Only the right onset location was activated for the LBBB whereas both right and left were activated for ALBBBm because in an LBBB the left bundle is not active.

3.2   Results

Table 1 shows the CV before the parameter estimation, after the LBBB parameter estimation and after the ALBBB parameter estimation. First, all Purkinje CV are higher than myocardial CV which is to be expected. We can see that the myocardial cells CV (as for the right Purkinje) is very similar between the LBBB and the ALBBB estimations. For the left Purkinje, we found 0.49 m/s for LBBB and 1.32 m/s for ALBBB, indicating that the model seems to identify the LBBB pathology (affected LP system). Moreover, the MC CV values lie in the myocardial CV range found in the literature [1]. The RP CV (as well as the LP CV for the ALBBB) is close to the Purkinje CV range found in the literature.

Figure 3 shows the simulation results after parameter estimation. Figure 3(a) represents the true (black) and simulated (blue) 12-lead ECG for the LBBB case and Fig. 3(b) the corresponding cardiac activation map. We can see that the shape of the ECG is coherent with the ground truth and especially the clear notched R wave on leads V5 and V6, indicator of an LBBB pathology. Figure 3(c) and (d) depict the results for the ALBBB, where both QRS on ECG and activation times are shorter than for the LBBB. The real and simulated ECG for ALBBB have similar shapes even though we can notice the notched V2 and V3 R waves (so RV and LV are not perfectly synchronous). It may indicate that our Purkinje zone delimitation could be improved.

4   Discussion

We showed a promising non-invasive parameter estimation and identified the activation of the Purkinje system. The fact that the RP and LP conductions are smaller than the literature range may be because we model the Purkinje system as a layer (not a small fiber network). For consistency reasons, we initialized the LBBB with only the right onset. However, it leads to different initial settings between ALBBB and LBBB parameter estimation. That is why we also ran the ALBBB using only the right onset: we found a similar myocardial CV (0.39 m/s), a higher left Purkinje CV (2 m/s) and a smaller right Purkinje (0.17 m/s). It seems that the model is compensating the absence of left onset, while still showing a clear left Purkinje activation. We have tested the sensitivity of our method

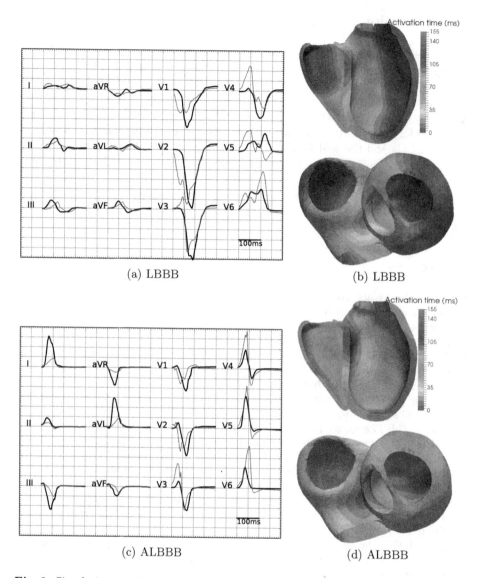

(a) LBBB

(b) LBBB

(c) ALBBB

(d) ALBBB

Fig. 3. Simulation results after parameter estimation. *LBBB:* (a) Real 12-lead ECG (black) and estimated (blue) during the 200 ms after onset activation. (b) Estimated activation map. *ALBBB:* (c) Real 12-lead ECG (black) and estimated (blue) during the 200 ms after onset activation. (d) Estimated activation map (Color figure online).

to the locations of the 9 torso electrode by adding Gaussian noise. After 5 tests with a perturbation mean of 7.5 mm in a random direction for each electrode, the relative differences to the estimated CVs have a mean of 3% (max = 10%). We can conclude that our method seems to be stable to small perturbations.

5   Conclusion

We have shown a method for estimating the activation of the left and right Purkinje system of the EP cardiac model based on the 12-lead ECG. The estimation of CV parameters for LBBB and absence of LBBB (same patient) shows a good agreement for the myocardium CV (0.39 m/s for ABBB, 0.40 m/s for LBBB), while the estimation of the left Purkinje CV seems to identify the pathology (1.32 m/s for ALBBB, 0.49 m/s for LBBB). Moreover, the plots of the simulated 12-lead ECGs and the real ECGs indicate similar shapes. We believe this work to be an interesting first step for understanding and modelling BBB pathology.

Acknowledgments. The research leading to these results has received funding from the Seventh Framework Programme (FP7/2007-2013) under grant agreement VP2HF n°611823.

References

1. Durrer, D., et al.: Total excitation of the isolated human heart. Circulation **41**, 899–912 (1970). Am Heart Assoc
2. Lorange, M., et al.: A computer heart model incorporating anisotropic propagation. J. Electrocardiol. **26**, 263–277 (1993). Elsevier
3. Potse, M., et al.: Similarities and differences between electrocardiogram signs of left bundle-branch block and left-ventricular uncoupling. In: Europace, vol. 14, pp. v33–v39. Eur Heart Rhythm Assoc (2012)
4. Zettinig, O., et al.: Data-driven estimation of cardiac electrical diffusivity from 12-lead ECG signals. Med. Image Anal. **18**, 1361–1376 (2014). Elsevier
5. Chávez, C.E., Zemzemi, N., Coudière, Y., Alonso-Atienza, F., Álvarez, D.: Inverse problem of electrocardiography: estimating the location of cardiac ischemia in a 3D realistic geometry. In: van Assen, H., Bovendeerd, P., Delhaas, T. (eds.) FIMH 2015. LNCS, vol. 9126, pp. 393–401. Springer, Heidelberg (2015). doi:10.1007/978-3-319-20309-6_45
6. Groth, A., Weese, J., Lehmann, H.: Robust left ventricular myocardium segmentation for multi-protocol MR. In: SPIE Medical Imaging, p. 83142S. International Society for Optics and Photonics (2012)
7. Mitchell, C., Schaeffer, D.: A two-current model for the dynamics of cardiac membrane. Bull. Math. Biol. **65**, 767–793 (2003). Springer, Heidelberg
8. Delingette, H., Ayache, N.: Soft tissue modeling for surgery simulation. In: Handbook of Numerical Analysis, vol. 12, pp. 453–550 (2004). Elsevier
9. Hansen, N.: The CMA evolution strategy: a comparing review. In: Lozano, J.A., Larrañaga, P., Inza, I., Bengoetxea, E. (eds.) Towards a New Evolutionary Computation. Studies in Fuzziness and Soft Computing, vol. 192, pp. 75–102. Springer, Heidelberg (2006)

4D Automatic Centre Detection of the Right and Left Ventricles from Cine Short-Axis MRI

Hakim Fadil[✉], John J. Totman, and Stephanie Marchesseau

Clinical Imaging Research Centre, A*STAR-NUS, Singapore, Singapore
dnrmhf@nus.edu.sg

Abstract. Segmentation of the heart ventricles from short axis Cine MRI is an active area of research. However, most of the solutions offered to radiologists are still semi-automatic. Several commercial software require from the users to input the centres of the ventricles for every image to segment which is fastidious and time-consuming. The automatic detection of these centres is challenging, especially, in the case of the right ventricle (RV). The variability in image quality, heart shape, thickness and motion, have led researchers to make assumptions not always valid regarding its position, blood pool intensity or shape. We aim in this work to offer a fast automatic, robust and accurate solution to this issue. By using the motion, and the pixel intensity, we are able to localize, recognize and select centres for both ventricles. First, our approach focuses on performing a coarse segmentation of each ventricle at the basal slice at the end-diastolic frame. The coarse segmentation of the left ventricle (LV) is then propagated to the following frames and below slices to reduce the region of interest. The greater reliability of the LV centre detection allows its use to define an area of search for the RV. We tested our method on 32 patients from the MICCAI 2012 RVSC Test1 and Test2 datasets and 10 volunteers, totalling 7485 images. We achieved a 99.3% success detection rate in the case of the LV, and 89.8% for the RV. We also show how the LV centre detection can be applied to define the LV central axis, and used to detect and correct misaligned slices.

Keywords: Centre detection · Left ventricle · Right ventricle · Alignment · Central axis

1 Introduction

The segmentation of the ventricles of the heart remains an active area of medical image analysis. It is of key interest to radiologists who use the results to evaluate the cardiac function. Many fully automatic solutions have been presented in the literature for the left ventricle (LV) [5], and the right ventricle (RV) [6]. However, most of the tools available to clinicians are semi-automatic and require manual input. This manual input is usually required for every image and, therefore, represents a tedious task prone to observer variability.

© Springer International Publishing AG 2017
T. Mansi et al. (Eds.): STACOM 2016, LNCS 10124, pp. 143–151, 2017.
DOI: 10.1007/978-3-319-52718-5_16

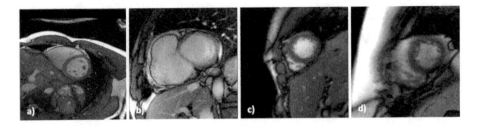

Fig. 1. Examples of short-axis slices illustrating the variability between images in terms of (i) image quality ($a \neq d$), (ii) RV shape ($a \neq b$), (iii) respective position ($a \neq c$) and (iv) contrast ($d \neq c$).

In this paper, we focus on the automatic detection of the centres of the ventricles. Localizing the centres of the ventricles will remove the need for manual input in commercial software such as Segment Medviso[1], CMR tools from Cardiovascular Imaging Solutions[2] or Circle Cardiovascular Imaging[3]. Additionally, the centres are necessary to define the LV central axis. From the LV central axis, 3D reconstruction can be performed after realignment of the short axis slices. Moreover, LV central axis and RV centres allow the definition of the 17 AHA zones for regional measurements.

The automatic detection of these centres is challenging, especially, in the case of the RV. Despite the variability in image quality, heart shape, thickness as illustrated in Fig. 1, current methods make assumptions such as [7] on the respective position, or [2] on the intensity profile, which remains difficult to predict because of the blood flow, the fat, and the trabeculations. We tackle this centre detection without these assumptions by a coarse-to-fine approach to detect the centre of each ventricle in every single image of a 4D sequence.

The proposed method was tested on 32 patients from the MICCAI 2012 RVSC Test1 and Test2 datasets and 10 volunteers. We also present an application of the LV centre detection algorithm to realign misaligned short-axis slices.

2   Methods

The proposed method uses motion and pixel intensity to detect, recognize, and select centres for both ventricles. First, the heart is located and cropped by estimating the motion throughout the frames at the basal slice. Then, a coarse segmentation of each ventricles is performed at the basal slice at the end-diastolic (ED) frame. The segmented LV is then propagated through the slices and frames to reduce the area of search. The LV centres are used to define a region of interest for the RV. The pipeline is illustrated in Fig. 2.

---

[1] http://medviso.com/products/segment/.

[2] http://www.cmrtools.com/.

[3] http://www.circlecvi.com/.

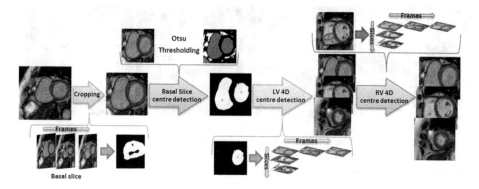

Fig. 2. Pipeline for 4D automatic centre detection. First, a cropping is performed on the 4D image. Then at the basal slice, both ventricles are detected, recognized and centres are selected. The result of this detection is then used to search in the 4D volume the centres of the LV. Finally, the LV centres are used to define elliptic areas of search around the RV centres.

2.1 Cropping

The first step of the proposed coarse-to-fine approach consists in cropping the image to delimit the heart. This will help in the detection by preventing possible false positives, and also reduce the overall computational time. The cropping method is first used on the basal slice. The basal slice is selected manually, as the first slice where the ventricles are the biggest and form a full ring (for instance Fig. 3a). However, automatic selection will be considered in the future using recently published method [4].

This cropping method is quite similar to the heart localization approach presented in [2], as we look for the region presenting most of the motion in the image. To observe the motion, we compute the sum of the absolute pixel-wise difference between 2 images of the cardiac cycle:

$$I_\Delta = \sum_{t=2}^{N} |I_1 - I_t|$$

where I_t is the 2D image representing the basal slice at time t.

The effect of the background noise is reduced by summing the absolute difference between the first frame and the following frames. Moreover, the small motions are attenuated by smoothing I_Δ with a Gaussian kernel (choosing a large σ to reduce the amount of noise). Otsu's thresholding algorithm is then applied to approximate the shape of the heart (Fig. 3), which may contain surrounding objects. The bounding box is defined as the smallest window W containing every pixel of the mask. In order to make up for possible errors W's size is increased by 5 pixels in every directions. The bounding box defined at the basal slice is then used for all the slices.

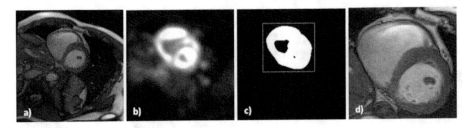

Fig. 3. Illustration of the cropping step. (a) Original image (size 192×192). (b) The smoothed I_Δ. (c) Otsu's binarization with in red the bounding box. (d) The result of the cropping (size 94×88). (Color figure online)

2.2   Centre Detection at Basal Slice

The ventricles are the most filled with blood in the ED frame, where they appear as big structures with high intensity. At that specific time, the ventricles can easily be discriminated from the background by using a thresholding method. In the literature, Otsu's model has been used for the same purpose [7].

The result obtained is an approximation of the blood pool of the ventricles, on which is applied a morphological reconstruction [3] to fill the holes present in all connected components and remove small papillary muscles.

The previously computed I_Δ is then used to reduce the number of potential ventricles. Only the 3 largest connected components sharing pixels with I_Δ are kept as illustrated in Fig. 4. We identify the LV as being the object with the highest circularity measure C [1] defined as $C = \dfrac{4\pi A}{P^2}$ where P is the perimeter, and A the area. The centre of the LV is chosen as the barycentre of the object and denoted LV_c.

The RV is then estimated between the two other objects Ω_1, Ω_2, by optimising the following function

$$\max_{\Omega_1, \Omega_2} \left[\frac{C_{\Omega_i}}{max(C_{\Omega_1}, C_{\Omega_2})} + \frac{|\Omega_i|}{max(|\Omega_1|, |\Omega_2|)} - \frac{dist(\Omega_i - LV_c)}{max(dist(\Omega_1 - LV_c), dist(\Omega_2 - LV_c))} \right]$$

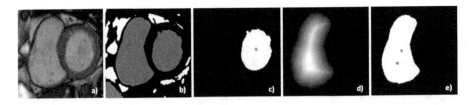

Fig. 4. (a) Original basal slice. (b) Otsu's binarization, in colours the 3 connected components kept. (c) The LV extracted with its centre (green star). (d) RV's distance map. (e) The RV extracted with its chosen centre (red star), and its barycentre (blue star). (Color figure online)

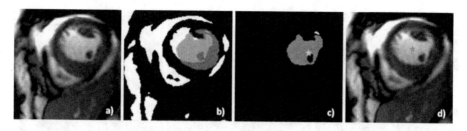

Fig. 5. (a) Original image. (b) The LV extracted at the previous slice (in green) is intersected with the result of Otsu on the original image. (c) The result of the intersection. In yellow, the centre of the previous slice, and in green the LV segmentation chosen for this slice. (d) The result of the detection in green. (Color figure online)

The largest and closest object to the LV with the highest circularity measure is selected. The centre of the RV is chosen as the maximum of the distance map (Fig. 4d and e) to account for the potential presence of fat and the non-circular shape of the RV, that will misplace the barycentre.

2.3   Left Ventricle Centre Detection on the 4D Sequence

To detect the centre of the other slices and frames, the area of search is reduced to allow faster computation, to prevent false positive due to fat tissue around the heart and to take into account the muscle narrowing toward the apex. Both the coarse segmentation of the LV and the detected centre (Fig. 4c) from the basal slice at ED are used to detect the LV centre of first the other slices and then the other frames of the cardiac cycle. First, for each new slice, Otsu's binarization is performed and intersected with the coarse mask from the previous slice, as described Fig. 5b. This intersection may contain several disconnected objects (Fig. 5c) from which the LV is detected as the object containing, or closest to, the LV centre from the previous slice. The centre of this LV is then defined as the barycentre of the selected coarse object (Fig. 5d).

To detect the centre of the LV for the other time frames, a similar process is applied using the coarse LV masks and the LV centres detected at ED. However, instead of performing Otsu on the whole image, it is only applied on the intersection with the coarse mask in order to give an apriori localization of the blood pool at end-systole (ES). Using the same ED inputs for all time frames allows parallel computing.

2.4   Right Ventricle Centre Detection on the 4D Sequence

Even more importantly for the RV, the area of search needs to be reduced to prevent the risk of detecting fat tissue which presents brighter intensity and sharper contrast than the very thin RV muscle. Similarly to the LV, the centre detection is first performed on all slices at ED, then on the other time frames of

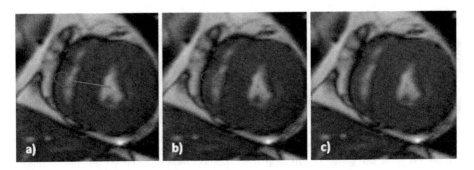

Fig. 6. From left to right. (a) Definition of the ellipse. (b) Binarization of the inside of the ellipse. (c) The selected centres.

the cardiac cycle. Due to the reliability of the LV detection, the LV centre can be used as a landmark to define the area of search in which the RV blood pool is assumed to be found. First, an ellipse is defined around the RV centre obtained from the previous slice at ED. Based on geometrical observations, the main axis size is set to a fourth of the distance between the current LV centre and the previous RV centre, and the minor axis size is set to a sixth of this distance (Fig. 6a). The ellipse is assumed to follow the narrowing of the RV towards the apex, and its motion during contraction. Otsu's algorithm is once again used to differentiate the blood pool from the background within the ellipse (Fig. 6b). Similarly to LV detection, the RV is chosen as the closest object to the centre of the ellipse and its barycentre defined as the centre of the RV for the current slice. The ellipses defined at ED are used to detect the RV centre in the other frames of the cardiac cycle, which allows parallel computing.

3 Results

We evaluated our algorithm on 32 patient short-axis volumes from the Test1 and Test2 datasets of the MICCAI 2012 RVS challenge [6] acquired on a Siemens Symphony Tim 1.5T MRI, and 10 volunteer scans acquired on a Siemens 3T Prisma. In total, the algorithm has been tested on 7485 images. The cropping is done on average in 65 ms, the detection on the basal slice (all frames) in 250 ms, and the detection on a slice (all frames) in 110 ms. The overall time for a 4D detection of 1 subject is less than 2 s. The tests were done on a Intel Xeon CPU ES-1650 3.20 GHz (12 cores). The detection is considered as successful if the centre is detected in the middle for the LV, and in the blood pool for the RV. Examples of successful detection are shown in the first row of the Fig. 7, for 2 apical and 2 basal slices.

The algorithm performs extremely well for the LV with a 99.3% success rate for all the patients, and a mean of 99.4% per patient. The failed detection happens only when the blood pool is not visible anymore due to the contraction. As for the RV, we achieved a satisfying 89.8% success rate over the 7485 images.

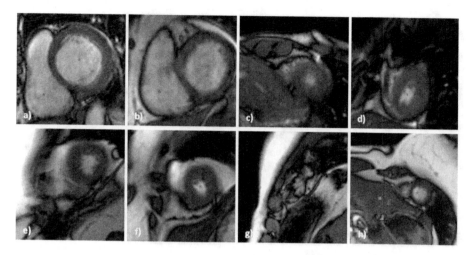

Fig. 7. Example results of the centre detector for the LV (green) and RV (red). (Color figure online)

There are several reasons to be considered for the 10% failures, Fig. 7 second row illustrates some of them.

In some cases, the presence of fat or fluid around the wall may be detected as part of the blood pool, especially, close to the apex at ES (Fig. 7e). Similarly to the LV, it might fail when the ventricle is completely closed by the contraction which usually happens around the apex at ES as shown in Fig. 7f. Overall, most of the errors are close to the apical slice, the algorithm fails to follow the sudden narrowing of the heart ventricles (Fig. 7g and h). Future improvements will consider a linear interpolation of the distance between the RV and LV centres to redefine the area of search towards the apex, and hopefully decrease the error rate.

3.1   LV Central Axis and Alignment

Misaligned slices are a frequent issue in short axis Cine MRI due to different breath-hold positions. In order to detect and correct the misaligned slices, we propose to use the LV central axis. The LV central axis is defined as the line joining the LV centre of the basal slice and the apex. To estimate the misalignment, the distance between the LV centre of each intermediates slices and the axis is computed. Then, Tukey's boxplot method [8] is used to detect the outliers among the set of distances. The outliers are considered as misaligned slices, and the translations needed to align them is calculated and applied. In our example, two iterations of the LV centre detection and alignment algorithm was needed to perfectly align the slices as shown in Fig. 8. This alignment method can only be efficient for a small number of misaligned slices. Aligning short-axis slices allows to perform 3D reconstruction of the LV geometry for further analysis such as motion tracking.

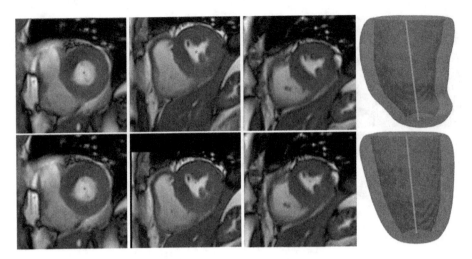

Fig. 8. First row: results of LV detector on misaligned slices, the middle image is clearly misaligned. Second row: results of the alignment algorithm, the middle image is perfectly aligned with the other slices. Last column illustrates on top a LV misaligned, and in the bottom a LV after alignment, the blue line represents the central axis. (Color figure online)

4 Discussion and Conclusion

The segmentation of ventricles in cine MRI is a challenging task due to the large variability in shape, motion, and image quality. Especially, in the case of the RV where, to the best of our knowledge, no robust automatic method has been made available to clinicians. We aimed through this work at presenting a robust technique for ventricle centre detection in 4D. Our goal is to simplify the traditional usage of segmentation tools by replacing the manual input required from clinicians. Our solution was tested on a database of 7485 images, presenting a large variability, in heart sizes, image quality, presence of artefact, and motion.

The LV centre detector showed close to 100% success rate, which makes it extremely reliable as an add-on to any semi-automatic tool directed to clinicians. Moreover, its precision allows us to use it to define the LV central axis. This central axis can be useful to detect and correct misalignment but also for 3D LV models and AHA regional segments definition. The results of RV detector were also satisfying as they reached the 90% threshold and represent, therefore, a usable solution to initialize a centre-based automatic segmentation method.

Acknowledgement. This work has been partially funded by the NMRC NUHS Centre Grant Medical Image Analysis Core (NMRC/CG/013/2013).

References

1. Jiang, L., Ling, S., Li, Q.: Fully automated segmentation of left ventricle using dual dynamic programming in cardiac cine MR images. In: SPIE Medical Imaging. International Society for Optics and Photonics (2016)
2. Atehortúa Labrador, A.M., Zuluaga, M.A., Ourselin, S., Giraldo, D., Romero Castro, E.: Automatic segmentation of 4D cardiac MR images for extraction of ventricular chambers using a spatio-temporal approach. In: SPIE Medical Imaging. International Society for Optics and Photonics (2016)
3. Lehmann, G.: Label object representation and manipulation with ITK. Insight J. **8** (2007)
4. Paknezhad, M., Marchesseau, S., Brown, M.S.: Automatic basal slice detection for cardiac analysis. In: SPIE Medical Imaging. International Society for Optics and Photonics (2016)
5. Petitjean, C., Dacher, J.-N.: A review of segmentation methods in short axis cardiac MR images. Med. Image Anal. **15**(2), 169–184 (2011)
6. Petitjean, C., Zuluaga, M.A., Bai, W., Dacher, J.-N., Grosgeorge, D., Jérôme Caudron, S., Ruan, I.B., Ayed, M.J., Cardoso, H.-C.C., et al.: Right ventricle segmentation from cardiac MRI: a collation study. Med. Image Anal. **19**(1), 187–202 (2015)
7. Ringenberg, J., Deo, M., Devabhaktuni, V., Berenfeld, O., Boyers, P., Gold, J.: Fast, accurate, and fully automatic segmentation of the right ventricle in short-axis cardiac MRI. Comput. Med. Imaging Graph. **38**(3), 190–201 (2014)
8. Tukey, J.W.: Box-and-whisker plots. In: Exploratory Data Analysis, pp. 39–43 (1977)

Novel Looped-Catheter-Based 2D-3D Registration Algorithm for MR, 3DRx and X-Ray Images: Validation Study in an Ex-vivo Heart

Michael V.N. Truong[1,2(✉)], Alison Liu[1], R. James Housden[1],
Graeme P. Penney[1], Mihaela Pop[2,3], and Kawal S. Rhode[1]

[1] Imaging Sciences and Biomedical Engineering, King's College London,
London, England, UK
{michael.truong,alison.liu,richard.housden,
graeme.penney,kawal.rhode}@kcl.ac.uk
[2] Physical Sciences, Sunnybrook Research Institute,
Sunnybrook Health Sciences Centre, Toronto, ON, Canada
mihaela.pop@utoronto.ca
[3] Department of Medical Biophysics, University of Toronto,
Toronto, ON, Canada

Abstract. In this paper, a novel 2D-3D cardiac image registration algorithm is proposed for application in X-ray-guided catheterisation procedures, and relies on a common technique of inserting a catheter and then looping it inside a chamber of the heart for visual reference. Registration starts with the isocentre-supine constraint and then iteratively refined by maximising a feature-based area metric using an inserted catheter loop and the segmented cardiac border from one or more X-ray views. Maximisation is done in two stages: first correcting for translational motion, and then simultaneously correcting for rotations and translations. The two-staged approach is demonstrated to be more accurate than a similar single-staged approach in an explanted porcine heart. In this experiment, accuracy was demonstrated to be within the 5-mm clinical requirement. On average, the algorithm could register images with a mean target registration error (TRE) of 4.6-mm when using two X-rays (biplane), and a mean reprojection distance (RPD) of 1.9 mm using a single view (monoplane).

Keywords: 2D-3D registration · Cardiac image registration · Image-guided procedures · MR · 3DRx · X-ray fluoroscopy · Biplane X-ray

1 Introduction

Catheter-based cardiac procedures, such as cardiac resynchronisation therapy [1], percutaneous coronary intervention [2] and RF ablation [3], require accurate and remote manipulation of catheters into the heart via an artery. These procedures are routinely guided under X-ray fluoroscopy due to its real-time imaging capabilities and excellent device visibility. Unfortunately, X-ray offers little soft-tissue contrast and no

© Springer International Publishing AG 2017
T. Mansi et al. (Eds.): STACOM 2016, LNCS 10124, pp. 152–162, 2017.
DOI: 10.1007/978-3-319-52718-5_17

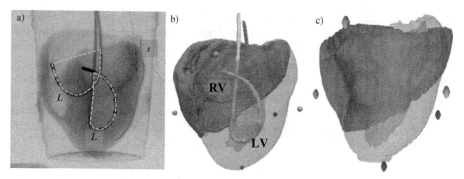

Fig. 1. Anterior view of a porcine heart in: (a) X-ray with catheter loops (*dashed yellow*) formed within their chambers and arc along the upper cardiac border (*solid red*); left (*translucent red*) and right (*blue*) ventricles surface renderings from (b) 3DRx and (c) MR scan segmentations. Five fiducial markers (*blue, red, green, orange, cyan*) used to obtain a gold standard registration were visible in each image modality. Catheters looped into the LV (*white*) and RV (*grey*) were in-place in both X-ray-based modalities but not in MR. (Color figure online)

depth information (Fig. 1a), making catheter navigation time-consuming and increases both the radiation exposure and the danger of perforating vessel walls [4, 5]. To mitigate these, it is desirable to overlay high soft-tissue-contrast 3D scans of the heart acquired from either CT, MR or 3D rotational X-ray (3DRx) [6–11] (Fig. 1b, c). However, the registration of such images is a challenging process. For instance, real-time registration can be performed accurately and automatically using a hybrid X-ray/MR guidance [6], but requires a dedicated hardware setup not widely available. One can use fiducial skin markers [7]; however, accuracy may be lost due to motion. The source of error due to motion can be avoided using anatomical features from the heart itself for registration [8]; unfortunately, repeat contrast agent injections may be needed for a reliable segmentation.

Alternatively, the use of the catheters for registration purposes has been recently explored, since they are the main instruments of the procedure and have excellent visibility in X-ray images while being placed directly into the heart [9–11]. In current clinical settings, a common registration technique involves inserting a catheter and looping it inside a chamber to provide a visual anchor for the interventionalist. Then, the preoperative 3D data from several X-ray views is manually aligned using a software platform such as EP navigator [10]. This technique was automated and its feasibility was previously explored in a phantom study [11], with the upper border of the cardiac shadow included as an additional constraint, as in [8]. The upper cardiac border is typically visible in X-ray and therefore avoids a contrast agent injection (Fig. 1a).

Biplanes help reduce out-of-plane errors associated with X-ray, but sequential acquisitions negatively affect the clinical workflow since the radiographer needs to rotate and then readjust the C-arm and the patient table, posing an issue for repeat registrations. Errors can also be caused by gating and catheter movements between images. These issues can be avoided using a simultaneous biplane fluoroscopy system [12]; however, these dedicated systems are expensive and not in widespread clinical use. On the other hand, single-view (monoplane) registration is advantageous where repeat registrations are required, for example, in case of bulk patient motion – a potential problem when the patient is sedated but not under general anaesthetics [6]. A single-view registration method could be used to detect when bulk patient motion has occurred and potentially correct a prior registration for this motion.

This paper aims to address these limitations and proposes a novel looped-catheter-based 2D-3D cardiac image registration algorithm. For evaluation, the algorithm is applied to an explanted pig heart model (Fig. 1a–c), where fiducial markers placed around the heart were used to help quantify the algorithm's accuracy. For clinical applicability, our target accuracy was 5 mm or better [5].

2 Method

The proposed 2D-3D registration algorithm is a feature-based approach that extends from [12] and designed to fit within the clinical workflow of an X-ray-guided catheter procedure. It relies on the formation of a catheter loop inside a target chamber of the heart as a constraining feature for registration, in addition to the upper cardiac border segmentation. The algorithm works with any number of X-ray views, and iteratively searches for the rigid-body transformation (RBT) M_{reg} that aligns preoperative 3D data projected onto X-ray images by maximising the metric $A = \sum_i \left(A^i_{\mathrm{loop}} - A^i_{\mathrm{border}} \right)$.

In each view, A^i_{loop} is the intersecting area between the catheter loop from the ith view and projections of the target chamber segmented from the preoperative 3D data, while A^i_{border} is the separation area between the upper border of the X-ray cardiac shadow and left (LV) and right ventricle (RV) projections segmented from the 3D data (Fig. 2).

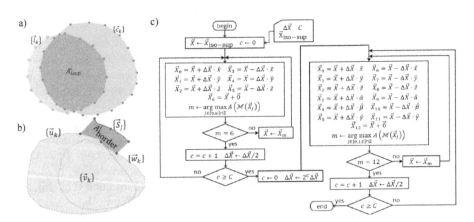

Fig. 2. (a) A_{loop} is the intersection (green) between the area within the catheter loop l (orange, orange circles) and target chamber's projection c^i (blue, blue circles). (b) Separation area A_{border} (purple) is between the X-ray cardiac border S^i (red line) and LV/RV polygon v^i (pink). (c) Flowchart of the $2 \times$ BNHC optimisation strategy used in the loop-catheter-based registration algorithm. (Color figure online)

2.1   Preoperative 3D and Intraoperative 2D Features for Constraint

Prior to catheterisation, a 3D scan of the heart is acquired followed by a semi-automatic segmentation of its chambers [13] to obtain points along the endocardial wall of the target chamber $C = \{\vec{C}_k\}$ and epicardial wall of the LV: $U = \{\vec{U}_k\}$ and RV: $W = \{\vec{W}_k\}$. Generally: $X = \{\vec{X}_k\}$ will be used to denote 3D point sets, and $X^i = \{\vec{X}^i_k\}$ for 2D point sets belonging to the ith view. The volumes of the segmented chambers and the numbers of vertices that make up the meshes after decimation are listed in Table 1.

Table 1. Summary of chamber segmentations with the blood pool (*b.p.*), myocardium (myo.) and total (*tot.*) volume V (cm^3), and the numbers of vertices (#) that make up their hulls.

Dataset	Modality	Target	Target chamber		LV			RV		
			b.p .V	#	tot. V	myo. V	#	tot. V	myo. V	#
Porcine heart	MR	LV	28.4	149	121.1	92.7	396	85.1	36.9	400
		RV	48.2	217						
	3DRx	LV	29.8	498	143.2	113.4	1379	78.9	28.7	998
		RV	50.2	740						

During the procedure, the heart should be at the isocentre of the X-ray system, with both the catheter loop, formed within the target chamber, and the upper cardiac shadow always in view. For each view, points are manually selected along the loop part of the catheter l^i and along the upper cardiac shadow S^i. Incomplete loops are closed with a straight line (Fig. 1a). Any number of X-rays can be used in the algorithm but each must be in the same cardiorespiratory phase as the preoperative acquisition, usually at end-diastole and end-respiration, when the heart is undergoing minimal motion. The 3D chamber features are brought into spatial correspondence via a perspective projection onto the X-ray views using camera matrices M^i [14]. For the target chamber, $c^i = M^i C$ and for the ventricles, $u^i = M^i U$ and $w^i = M^i W$. A summary of the catheter loop configurations and X-ray 2D images is listed in (Table 2).

Table 2. Summary of catheter loop configurations, and points picked along catheter loop and upper cardiac border in each X-ray view of the configuration. The number of points (#), encompassing area (A) and perimeter (p) are listed for the catheter loops, along with the number of points (#) and total linear arclength (l) of the border.

Dataset	Target	Configuration	View	Catheter loop			Border	
				#	A(mm^2)	p(mm)	#	l(mm)
Porcine heart	LV	DAo-LV	PA	12	290.1	82.7	12	67.7
			RAO 45°	14	494.7	94.4	17	85.8
	RV	SVC-RV	PA	12	1030.2	128.2	12	67.7
			RAO 45°	10	843.3	114.4	17	85.8

2.2   Area-Based Metric for Each View

The positive part of the metric A_{loop} measures how much of the catheter loop is contained within the projection of the target chamber in each X-ray view. To quantify this, convex hulls of the projected chamber c^i and of the catheter loop l^i are extracted using a fast radial sweep hull routine [15]. The intersecting polygon between the hulls are found using a general polygon clipping routine [16] and A_{loop}^i is the area of this polygon.

The negative part of the metric A_{border}^i measures the separation between the upper cardiac border in X-ray and combined LV/RV projections $v^i = u^i \cap w^i$ (Fig. 2b). To calculate this, the curve S^i and polygon vertices v^i are arranged in contiguous order and reparameterised by arclength. Then for each point in S^i, starting from the middle point, the nearest unique point in v^i is picked to form n^i, such that $|S^i| = |n^i|$. A_{border}^i is the area of the polygon whose vertices are $S^i \cup n^i$.

The metric is designed to be suitable for any number of X-ray views, although intuitively, the ideal views are the ones where the catheter loop encloses the largest area and closely matches the area of the projection of the target chamber (Fig. 1). This usually occurs in PA view since the points where the catheter enters and exits the chambers of the heart are almost in-plane. When the loop is viewed from other angles, its minor axis decreases, resembling a flattened ellipse. In these cases, the catheter loop still provides two points of constraints. Fitting the loop inside the chamber represents a circular constraint that could lead to large rotational errors when registering. The inclusion of the upper cardiac border adds a constraint to minimise this free rotation.

2.3   Iterative Search Strategy

In order to align the 2D and 3D data, the algorithm starts with an initial guess RBT using the isocentre and supine constraint $M_0(\vec{X}) \leftarrow M_{\text{IS}}$, and then incrementally changes the three translational and three rotational degrees of freedom $\vec{X} = (x, y, z, \theta, \phi, \psi)$ until the area-based metric is maximised: $J = \text{argmax}_j A(\vec{X}_j)$, $M_{\text{reg}} = M_J$ (Fig. 2c).

The algorithm makes incremental changes $\Delta \vec{X}$ using the *best neighbour hill climbing* (BNHC) approach as previously described in [11], undergoing 15 rounds of iteration with each component of $\Delta \vec{X}$ decreasing by half after each iteration. In many cases, the supine constraint may provide a good initial estimate for the rotational parameters of M_{reg}, since the patient usually lies on the table bed in the same, repeatable way. However, depending on the individual case, the heart may not lie at the exact isocentre of the imaging systems, and therefore, there may be a large translational error between the images after applying the isocentre-supine constraint. In these cases, it is assumed better to first find the translational components of $\vec{X}$ before finding the rotational ones as this may increase the efficiency of the optimisation in terms of speed and accuracy, since the initial, large translational error can be corrected first without having to spend time considering potentially erroneous rotational corrections. Thus, in this paper, a variation of the BNHC method is constructed which first finds the translational components of M_{reg} using the same iteration and stopping criteria as the BNHC method described above. Then, the algorithm starts to search through the entire set of parameters of $\Delta\vec{X}$. This modification will be referred as the two-staged BNHC (2 × BNHC), while the former is referred to as the one-staged BNHC (1 × BNHC). A flowchart of the 2 × BNHC is shown in Fig. 2c.

2.4   Ex vivo Imaging Experiment Using an Explanted Porcine Heart

To validate the proposed registration algorithm, an *ex vivo* experiment was designed to emulate the workflow of a typical cardiac catheterization. In this study an explanted biventricular healthy porcine heart, previously preserved in formalin and with the atria removed. The heart was securely placed in a plastic jar, with five ECG chest electrodes glued onto the jar as fiducial markers visible in both MR and X-ray images. The jar was then imaged using a GE Signa Excite 1.5T MR scanner at a $0.55 \times 0.55 \times 2\text{-mm}^3$ voxel size with a spoiled gradient echo pulse sequence (NEX = 1, TE = 2.16 ms, TR = 10.18 ms, $\theta = 30°$). Subsequently, the jar was placed on an X-ray table equipped with a Innova 2121^{IQ}, GE Healthcare C-arm, followed by a 3DRx image acquisition (196° arc, 147 views, V_p = 60 kV, I = 97 mA). To reduce the streaking artefacts in the 3DRx, it was first smoothened with a 3^3 Gaussian kernel following a two-fold sub-sampling, for a final isotropic voxel size of $0.45 \times 0.45 \times 0.45 \text{ mm}^3$. While still on the X-ray table, catheters were looped into the LV and then the RV (Fig. 1a, b) followed by biplane acquisitions in PA and RAO 45° ($0.4 \times 0.4 \text{ mm}^2$ pixel size, SOD = 72 cm, SID = 119 cm) for each catheter configuration. If vessels and atria were still attached to the heart, the LV catheter would typically enter via the aorta and the RV catheter via the superior vena cava.

The LV and RV ventricular chambers of the volumes were then segmented [13]. For the MR, the segmented chamber volume of the LV was 28 mm^3 and of the RV was 48 mm^3. For 3DRx, these were 30 mm^3 and 50 mm^3 respectively (Table 1). From both biplane X-ray images of the heart, points along the looping catheter and upper border of the cardiac shadow were manually selected (Fig. 2a). The LV catheter loop enclosed an area of 290 mm^2 in PA and 495 mm^2 in RAO 45°. For the RV loop, these were 1030 mm^2 and 843 mm^2 respectively. The segmented upper cardiac border's arclengths were 68 mm and 86 mm in these views (Table 2).

2.5   Registration and Accuracy Assessment

Once all features were extracted, registration was performed between X-ray and MR and then between X-ray and 3DRx for both the LV and RV catheter loop configurations. The isocentre-supine constraint provided a starting point for the registration, which was then iteratively refined using both the 1x and 2xBNHC for comparison. $\Delta\vec{X}$ was (2 mm, 2 mm, 2 mm, 3.5°, 3.5°, 3.5°). The translational step sizes were 2 mm, being sufficiently larger than the image resolution, and the angular step sizes were 3.5° as this is the rotation needed for a 10-cm diameter heart to have at least 2-mm displacement at its epicardial border. For each catheter-modality configuration, both optimising strategies were performed three times: (i) using biplane X-ray views, (ii) with the left view and (iii) with the right view; for a total of 24 registrations. To perform these, a custom software was written in C#.NET running on a Microsoft Windows 7 64-bit laptop equipped with a dual 3-GHz Intel Core 2 CPU and 4 GB of RAM.

The five fiducial markers were visible in MR, 3DRx and both X-ray views and were manually selected to provide independent X-ray-MR and X-ray-3DRx registrations with FREs of 1.47 mm and 1.65 mm respectively [14]. The accuracy of the registration M_{reg} was compared against the fiducial-marker-based registration M_{gold} which acted as a ground truth. When registering with biplane X-ray images, accuracy was assessed in terms of a mean 3D target registration error (TRE) which is averaged from the individual TREs of each vertex belonging to the segmentation of the regions of interest (Table 1). For single-view registration, accuracy was measured in terms of a mean reprojection distance (RPD), averaged over the same vertices. Both TRE and RPD are established measure of accuracy and therefor enables comparability with other registration algorithms [14].

3   Results

The 2D-3D image registration algorithm was applied to both looped-catheter configurations of the heart. Both 1xBNHC and 2xBNHC variations of the algorithms were run for comparison. *Accuracy* was assessed in terms of a mean 3D-TRE for biplane configurations and in terms of a mean RPD for monoplane configurations, measured over each ventricular chamber of the heart (RV/LV) and over the whole heart, respectively. The algorithm was used to register both MR and 3DRx scans of the heart onto PA and RAO 45° X-ray views, and in both biplane and monoplane modes, for a total of 24 registrations.

Accuracy of Registration. The isocentre-supine constraint provided an initial starting point for the algorithm with 13.0-mm mean 3D-TRE (WH) with respect to the gold standard. Registrations using the (first) LV catheter-loop configuration are shown as overlays in Fig. 3a–c with a spatial distribution of 3D-TRE over the heart. The 1 × BNHC yielded an average accuracy of 6.53-mm TRE while the 2 × BNHC yielded an average accuracy of 4.63 mm.

For monoplane registration, the isocentre-supine constraint started the registration with a 10.6-mm RPD, on average. The first looped-catheter-configuration overlays are shown in Fig. 3d–e, showing a spatial distribution of RPD over the heart and use the same colour scale for visual comparison across all 16 overlays. The 1 × BNHC yielded an average accuracy of 2.64-mm RPD while the 2 × BNHC yielded an average accuracy of 1.85 mm. Individual accuracies for both types of registration are listed in Table 3 below.

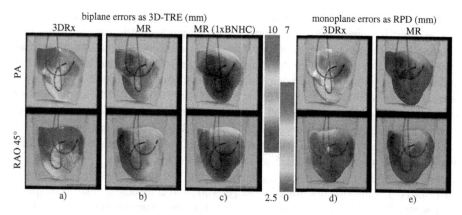

Fig. 3. Colour mapping of the 3D surface renderings show the spatial distribution of registration error overlaid on the X-ray in PA (top row) and RAO 45° (bottom row) views. Column (a, b, c) biplane 2xBNHC strategy applied to (a) 3DRx and (b) MR, and (c) 1xBNHC strategy applied to MR shown for comparison. (d) Monoplane 2xBNHC strategy is applied to 3DRx and (e) MR. Poor registration has a dominantly red colour. Colour bars are placed side-by-side for comparability. (Color figure online)

Table 3. Biplane and monoplane registration applied using isocentre-supine initialisation for $2 \times$ BNHC. Computational time (t) recorded along with the registration error over the ventricles of the heart (LV, RV) and over the whole heart (WH). For monoplane registration, results list average between PA and RAO 45° views. Results are then averaged over the four catheter-modality configurations and compared to $1 \times$ BNHC. Standard deviations are reported in brackets for the whole heart.

Configuration	Method	t(s)	Biplane registration error mean 3D-TRE (mm)			t(s)	Monoplane registration error mean RPD (mm)		
			LV	RV	WH		RV	RV	WH
Isocentre-supine	Initial		12.9	13.2	13.0		10.4	10.9	10.6
MR LV loop	$2 \times$ BNHC	45.4	4.8	5.0	4.7 (0.2)	31.7	2.1	2.7	2.5 (0.7)
MR RV loop	$2 \times$ BNHC	33.8	4.1	4.3	4.1 (0.2)	13.1	2.4	2.6	2.6 (0.5)
3DRx LV loop	$2 \times$ BNHC	32.4	4.4	5.5	4.9 (0.7)	21.9	1.0	1.6	1.2 (0.3)
3DRx RV loop	$2 \times$ BNHC	35.1	4.4	5.5	4.9 (0.7)	23.8	1.0	1.6	1.2 (0.3)
Average	$2 \times$ BNHC	36.7	4.4	5.1	4.6 (0.4)	22.6	1.6	2.1	1.9 (0.5)
Average	$1 \times$ BNHC	38.7	6.5	7.0	6.5 (0.4)	13.5	2.5	2.8	2.6 (0.8)

4 Discussion and Future Work

In this paper, a novel 2D-3D image registration algorithm was developed to overlay 3D MR and 3DRx data onto X-rays, using a looped catheter visible in fluoroscopy. Looping a catheter in a chamber of the heart as a constant visual anchor during an interventional procedure is a commonly used technique in clinical practice, and therefore would be a valid assumption. The algorithm was tested using an explanted porcine heart by mimicking a roadmap for catheter navigation in catheter-based procedures. The accuracy of the registration was assessed using a fiducial-marker-based gold standard. The algorithm used a local, iterative approach and therefore required an initial guess, in this case the isocentre-supine constraint. This provided, on average, starting accuracies of 13.0 mm TRE for biplane and 10.6 mm RPD for monoplane setups, which is not accurate enough for clinical applications [5]. However, the algorithm was able to improve accuracy within a mean TRE of 4.6 mm and a mean RPD of 1.9 mm (total average), with all four catheter-modality configurations achieving whole-heart accuracies within the 5-mm clinical tolerance.

For both mono- and biplane registrations, the two-staged strategy consistently performed better than the one-staged strategy, while still comparable in terms of speed, as presented in Table 1. One possible reason the two-staged approach is more accurate, is that the initial registration error due to the isocentre-supine constraint may contain larger translational components than angular components, leading to large adjustments in rotations, which may be an erroneous assumption by the optimising strategy. Another reason is that in the two-staged approach, when switching between the two stages, the increments are reset to the initial sizes of 2 mm/3.5°, commonly known as a *reset*. Resetting the optimisation has the benefit of escaping a local maximum if it was trapped in one.

Two catheter-loop configurations were tested, one large loop in the LV and a smaller, incomplete loop in the RV (Fig. 1a). The LV loop performed better than the RV, which may be the result of having a larger loop size (Table 2). The positive part of the metric relies on a good formation of the catheter loop where the catheter is in full contact with the chamber wall and also on the osculating plane of the loop being parallel to the X-ray imaging plane. When these are not the case, erroneous translations and rotations, can move the catheter loop towards the projected target chamber wall, without impacting the metric. One possible extension to this algorithm would be to include the ostia of the vessels from where the catheter enters and exits as additional constraints for registration. This would add two positions along the catheter that are guaranteed to be touching the wall and therefore help limit the range of movement the catheter can make in relation to the chamber.

The proposed method requires several manual-interaction steps: the catheter and heart boundaries need to be manually drawn on the fluoroscopic images, and the heart chambers needs to be semi-manually segmented from the 3D modality. However, there has been recent research which show promise towards automating these steps [17, 18]. A further improvement could be to introduce a multi-resolution search as in [19]. Using a fast low-resolution search could potentially provide a better initial guess than the isocentre-supine assumptions without significant computational overhead. On the other hand, a better initial guess could significantly speed up the algorithm due to a smaller search space.

Overall, the results of this novel registration algorithm look promising. The validation experiment using the explanted heart provided an ideal scenario to quantify the registration errors in the absence of motion artifacts; however, the study was limited to only one heart. Furthermore, while this study is more clinically realistic than a phantom study, the explanted heart is rigid and stationary. Thus, future work will address the potential errors due to cardiac and respiratory motion by applying the method to patient data. Noticeably, the reduced imaging requirement of single-view registration, compared to biplane registration, is ideal as it fits better with the clinical workflow. This is particularly well suited for correcting a prior registration affected by bulk patient motion, in which case the initial guess registration to start the local search is the prior registration instead of the supine-isocentre constraint. Single-view registration could also be used to detect if a prior registration has been compromised. In this case, the correction can be either performed immediately or flagged to the clinician for final decision.

References

1. Shea, J.B., Sweeney, M.O.: Cardiac resynchronization therapy: a patient's guide. Circulation **108**, e64–e66 (2003)
2. Holmes, D.R., Williams, D.O.: Catheter-based treatment of coronary artery disease. Contemp. Rev. Intervent. Cardiol. **1**, 60–73 (2008)
3. Lee, G., Sanders, P., Kalman, J.M.: Catheter ablation of atrial arrythmias: state of the art. Lancet **380**(9852), 1509–1519 (2012)
4. Lickfett, L., Mahesh, M., Vasamreddy, C., Bradley, D., Jayam, V., Eldadah, Z., Dickfeld, T.: Radiation exposure during catheter ablation of atrial fibrillation. Circulation **110**, 3003–3010 (2004)
5. Linte, C.A., Lang, P., Rettmann, M.E., Cho, D.S., Holmes III, D.R., Robb, R.A., Peters, T. M.: Accuracy considerations in image-guided cardiac interventions: experience and lessons learned. Int. J. Comput. Assist. Radiol. Surg. **7**, 13–25 (2011)
6. Rhode, K., Ma, Y., Housden, J., Karim, R., Razavi, R.: Clinical applications of image fusion for electrophysiology procedures. In: 9th IEEE ISBI, Barcelona, Spain (2012)
7. Gutiérrez, L.F., de Silva, R., Ozturk, C., Sonmez, M., Raman, V.K., Sachdev, V., Aviles, R. J., Waclawiw, M.A., McVeigh, E., Lederman, R.: Technology preview: X-ray fused with MRI during invasive cardiovascular procedures. Cathet. Cardiovasc. Interv. **70**, 773–882 (2007)
8. Daul, C., Lopen-Hernandez, J., Wolf, D., Karcher, G., Ethévenot, G.: 3-D multimodal cardiac data superimposition using 2-D image registration and 3-D reconstruction from multiple views. Image Vis. Comput. **27**, 790–802 (2009)
9. Truong, M., Gordon, T., Razavi, R., Penney, G., Rhode, Kawal, S.: Analysis of catheter-based registration with vessel-radius weighting of 3D CT data to 2D X-ray for cardiac catheterisation procedures in a phantom study. In: Camara, O., Konukoglu, E., Pop, M., Rhode, K., Sermesant, M., Young, A. (eds.) STACOM 2011. LNCS, vol. 7085, pp. 139–148. Springer, Heidelberg (2012). doi:10.1007/978-3-642-28326-0_14
10. Ma, Y., Duckett, S., Chinchapatnam, P., Gao, G., Sheety, A., Rinaldi, C.A., Schaeffter, T., Rhode, K.S.: MRI to X-ray fluroscopy overlay for guidance of cardiac resynchronization therapy procedures. In: Computing in Cardiology, Belftast, Northern Ireland, UK (2010)
11. Truong, M.V.N., Penney, G.P., Rhode, K.S.: Feasibility study of looped-catheter-based 2D-3D image registration of CT and X-Rays for cardiac catheterization procedures in a phantom experiment. In: Camara, O., Mansi, T., Pop, M., Rhode, K., Sermesant, M., Young, A. (eds.) STACOM 2012. LNCS, vol. 7746, pp. 317–325. Springer, Heidelberg (2013). doi:10.1007/978-3-642-36961-2_36

12. Pathak, C., Van Horn, M., Weeks, S., Bullitt, E.: Comparison of simultaneous and sequential two-view registration for 3D/2D registration of vascular images. In: MICCAI, Palm Springs, CA, USA (2005)
13. Zhang, H., Goodlett, C., Burke, T., Tustison, N.: ITK-SNAP, ITK-SNAP Team, 17 February 2011. www.itksnap.org. Accessed 10 12 2012
14. van de Kraats, E.B., Penney, G.P., et al.: Standardized evaluation methodology for 2-D–3-D registration. IEEE Trans. Med. Imaging 24(9), 1177–1189 (2005)
15. Sinclair, D.: S-hull; a fast sweep hull routine for Delauney triangulation 2010. www.s-hull.org
16. Johnson, A.: Clipper - an open source freeware polygon clipping library, 23 May 2013. http://www.angusj.com/delphi/clipper.php
17. Cazalas, M., Bismuth, V., Vaillant, R.: An image-based catheter segmentation algorithm for optimized electrophysiology procedure workflow. In: Ourselin, S., Rueckert, D., Smith, N. (eds.) FIMH 2013. LNCS, vol. 7945, pp. 182–190. Springer, Heidelberg (2013). doi:10. 1007/978-3-642-38899-6_22
18. Albà, X., Rosa, M., i Ventura, F., Lekadir, K., Tobon-Gomez, C., Hoogendoorn, C., Frangi, A.F.: Automatic cardiac LV segmentation in MRI using modified graph cuts with smoothness and interslice constraints. Magn. Reson. Med. 72(6), 1775–1784 (2013)
19. Xu, R., Athavale, P., Nachman, A., Wright, G.A.: Multiscale registration of real-time and prior MRI data for image-guided cardiac interventions. IEEE Trans. Biomed. Eng. 61(10), 2621–2632 (2014)

Left-Ventricle Basal Region Constrained Parametric Mapping to Unitary Domain

Antoni Gurgui[1]([✉]), Debora Gil[1,2], Vicente Grau[3], and Enric Marti[2]

[1] Computer Vision Center of Catalunya, Universitat Autonoma de Barcelona,
Barcelona, Spain
agurgui@cvc.uab.cat
[2] Computer Sciences Department, Universitat Autonoma de Barcelona,
Barcelona, Spain
[3] Department of Engineering Science, Institute of Biomedical Engineering,
University of Oxford, Oxford, UK

Abstract. Due to its complex geometry, the basal ring is often omitted when putting different heart geometries into correspondence. In this paper, we present the first results on a new mapping of the left ventricle basal rings onto a normalized coordinate system using a fold-over free approach to the solution to the Laplacian. To guarantee correspondences between different basal rings, we imposed some internal constrained positions at anatomical landmarks in the normalized coordinate system. To prevent internal fold-overs, constraints are handled by cutting the volume into regions defined by anatomical features and mapping each piece of the volume separately. Initial results presented in this paper indicate that our method is able to handle internal constrains without introducing fold-overs and thus guarantees one-to-one mappings between different basal ring geometries.

Keywords: Laplacian · Constrained maps · Parameterization · Basal ring

1 Introduction

Building statistical models (or atlases) of the heart is central for investigating and understanding tissue functions and properties. A main step in this direction is the definition of reference frames, or unitary domains, that allow to compare different geometries in a meaningful way. Ideally, these domains should assign equal coordinates to corresponding anatomical features and, at the same time, align the intermediate zones that might present different shapes (i.e. different trabeculae architectures).

The definition of cardiac atlases is an active field of research and several methods to put the geometries into correspondence and build atlases have been proposed [13,19]. Existing methods can be split into two main categories. Methods that deform a geometry to another one [7,12] and those that build a parametric description of the ventricular shapes, using basis functions like thin-plate

© Springer International Publishing AG 2017
T. Mansi et al. (Eds.): STACOM 2016, LNCS 10124, pp. 163–171, 2017.
DOI: 10.1007/978-3-319-52718-5_18

splines [2], hermite functions [11] or B-Splines [5], to define a mapping between different geometries. Recently, parameterizations using the solution to the Laplacian have been proposed to put cardiac surfaces into correspondence. In [14,16], a 3-step method to map the left ventricle cut at basal level onto a disk domain is proposed. A first unconstrained map is generated by solving the Laplacian with the boundary of the shape mapped to the boundary of the domain. Then, the apex is fixed to the center of the domain and a final parameterization if calculated using a quasi-conformal metric. Another example is presented in [10], where constraints for the atrial surface mapping are imposed by defining boundary conditions inside the domain.

However, most of the methods rely on a simplified geometry of the heart at the basal region, using a flat "top" and discarding the basal ring due to its complex shape. A main concern in cutting the geometry using a short axis plane to build cardiac models is the uncertainty of cutting possible connectivity of cardiac muscular architecture [15]. Although such connectivity has not been rigorously proved, several works [1,6] support the importance of fiber orientation in electromechanical simulations of the heart and, thus, we believe that basal connectivity should be explored. We propose to use the solution to Laplacian in order to define coordinates over the basal region of the left ventricle (LV). This enables to take this region into account when comparing different LV volumes. To this end, we propose to map the left ventricular basal structure to a normalized coordinate domain imposing some inner fixed positions on certain anatomical landmarks that are extended over the rest of the volume.

In this study we investigate the definition of a volumetric left ventricular base reference frame with constrained coordinates at some anatomical features, or places, based on the discrete mesh Laplacian presented in [17] and defining interior fixed coordinates as in [8]. This method presents the following advantages: allows to handle arbitrary polygonal constraints, can be extended to other organ geometries and it is easy to implement and reproduce.

2   Materials and Methods

To develop the method we have used the normal hearts from John Hopkins Canine Hearts database[1] [9]. This database consists of *ex-vivo* magnetic resonance image (MRI) volumes of canine hearts. More precisely, to focus on the basal ring, we studied the SA slices comprising the 35% (i.e. regions 1–6 of the AHA division [3]) of the left ventricle (LV) volume. We generated the initial volumetric meshes defining a vertex for each voxel and their connectivity from their 26-adjacency in the image.

To constrain interior coordinates, anatomical features and extracted geometric landmarks were fixed. Anatomical features include the basal ring, the endocardium and the epicardium. Geometric landmarks consist of medial surface of the volumes [18], the boundaries between interoseptal and inferoseptal and between inferolateral and anterolateral basal regions (see Fig. 1).

---

[1] Avaliable at: http://cvrgrid.org/data/ex-vivo.

2.1 Left Ventricle Volume Parameterization Using Laplacian Solution

Laplacian operators [4] are powerful mathematical tools that allow to define coordinate systems on manifolds, or volumes, with values fixed at some locations. These fixed values are called boundary conditions (BC) and can be coordinates constraints (Dirichlet BC) or derivative constraints (Neumann BC). When defining coordinate systems, Dirichlet conditions allow to constraint specific coordinates to specific locations, which are then extended by the solution of the Laplacian over the whole domain. This also implies that their setting is central to put different geometries into correspondence.

Given a 3D mesh $\mathcal{M}$ extracted from an MRI volume, we propose to obtain a parameterization from the Cartesian space to our defined 3D unitary domain $\mathcal{D} = [0,1] \times [0,1] \times [0.65,1]$ (see Fig. 1) using the 3 coordinate functions. We use a similar nomenclature as spherical coordinates and name our three unitary domain coordinates radius r for the depth coordinate ranging from endocardium to epicardium, angular θ for a circumferential coordinate defined in short axis (SA) and elevation φ for a coordinate defined in SA along the basal part of the left ventricles. Mathematically, we want to define a mapping between our mesh $\mathcal{M}$ to the unitary domain $\mathcal{D}$:

$$\mathbb{R}^3 \supset \mathcal{M} \to \mathcal{D} \subset \mathbb{R}^3$$
$$(x, y, z) \to (r, \theta, \varphi)$$

To obtain this mapping, we use the solution to the Laplacian to define each coordinate:

$$\left.\begin{array}{l} 1.\ \Delta r = 0 \text{ with } r|_{\mathcal{M}_r} = r_C \\ 2.\ \Delta\theta = 0 \text{ with } \theta|_{\mathcal{M}_\theta} = \theta_C \\ 3.\ \Delta\varphi = 0 \text{ with } \varphi|_{\mathcal{M}_\varphi} = \varphi_C \end{array}\right\} \tag{1}$$

for Δ the Laplacian operator, M_r, $\mathcal{M}_\theta$, $\mathcal{M}_\varphi$ the specific anatomical sites in the 3D mesh $\mathcal{M}$ where the values of each coordinate, r, θ, φ are constrained, respectively, to $r_C := r_C(x, y, z)$, $\theta_C = \theta_C(x, y, z)$ and $\varphi_C = \varphi_C(x, y, z)$.

As our domains are discrete meshes obtained from MRI volumes, we use the discrete Laplace operator to compute solutions to (1). By the mean value Theorem [4], solutions to Eq. (1) can be approximated by the following 3 linear systems (one for each coordinate):

$$1.\ Ar = b_R; \quad 2.\ A\theta = b_\theta; \quad 3.\ A\varphi = b_\varphi \tag{2}$$

with A a sparse matrix defined from the triangulation adjacency, the size of A being $N_v x N_v$ with N_v the number of mesh vertices [3] and b the independent term given by the boundary conditions evaluated at each anatomical site (M_r, $\mathcal{M}_\theta$, $\mathcal{M}_\varphi$). If $N(i)$ is the 1-ring of V_i defined as the n adjacent voxels in the volume, then A is given by:

$$A = \begin{cases} 1 & \text{if } j \in N(i), \ i \neq j \\ 0 & \text{if } j \notin N(i), \ i \neq j \\ -\sum_{k \neq i} a_{ik} & \text{if } i = j \end{cases} \tag{3}$$

Given that the matrix A is the same for the 3 coordinates and only depends on the mesh connectivity defined by the MRI volume, the only thing that remains to be defined are boundary conditions b_r, b_θ and b_φ and their corresponding anatomical meshes.

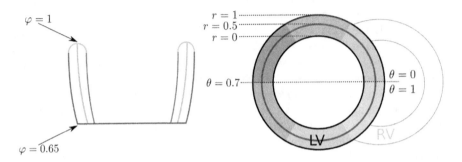

Fig. 1. Schematic description of fixed landmarks and their values in $\mathcal{D}$. Left: vertical long axis view, with the upper surface in light blue, the lowest plane in dark blue, the endocardium in green, the epicardium in red and the medial surface in grey. Right: SA view with colored AHA basal regions. (Color figure online)

2.2 Constrained Coordinates for the Left Ventricle

The fixed coordinates were defined using the following anatomical structures used by clinicians: the basal ring, the endocardium and the epicardium. The SA cut defining the lower boundary of the basal region was also considered to complete its boundary. Moreover, to demonstrate the capacity of the method to constrain interior boundaries, and have a better definition of the radial and elevation coordinates at the basal part, we have extracted the medial surface of each volume, as defined in [18]. In Fig. 2 we show these landmarks with respect to the volume. These anatomical landmarks are used to define boundary conditions for each coordinate as follows.

The values of some coordinates are well defined on some of the sites, like radius equal 0 at endocardium and equal 1 at epicardium. However, it is not so straightforward to extend such values to the complete basal region. We propose to use the Laplacian for surfaces to extend the values that are easily identified to the whole basal ring boundary (endocardium, epicardium, SA lower cut and basal region upper surface) to define the boundary functions for each coordinate. Such boundary functions will be used to obtain the coordinate value inside the whole volume solving each of the systems in (2).

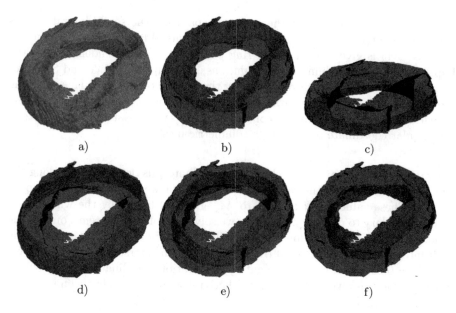

Fig. 2. Examples of segmentations masks: (a) whole volume, (b) upper surface, (c) lower plane, (d) epicardium, (e) medial surface and (f) endocardium

Radial Coordinate. The radial coordinate $r \in [0,1]$ normalizes the width of the basal region and, thus, it should be set to $r = 0$ at the endocardium and $r = 1$ at the epicardium. To obtain a more accurate transition we force an additional interior constraint at the medial surface with $r = 0.5$. Therefore, the anatomical mesh $\mathcal{M}_r$ is given by endocardium, epicardium, basal ring, SA lower plane and the medial surface. The boundary function b_r is obtained from the values fixed at endocardium, epicardium and medial surface as follows.

We extend the radial coordinate over the basal ring upper surface and lowest SA plane of the volume ((Fig. 2b and c), respectively), using the solutions to the Laplacian for each surface (basal ring and SA cut). For each surface, the matrix A in (3) is computed using the connectivity given by their masks in the MRI volume. As boundary conditions, we set $r = 0$ in the intersection of each surface with the endocardium, $r = 0.5$ in the intersection with the medial surface and $r = 1$ in the intersection with the epicardium.

Angular Coordinate. The angular coordinate θ is the circumferential coordinate defined in SA along the volume, counterclockwise positive defined. This coordinate allows the unfolding of the LV as shown in Fig. 1. To define its origin $\theta = 0$ we have used the boundary between basal interoseptal and basal inferoseptal regions defined by the American Heart Association (AHA). At the same time, we have fixed $\theta = 0.7$ in the boundary between basal inferolateral and basal anterolateral regions. Although the "natural" coordinate value should be 0.5, we forced it to 0.7 to show the effect of fixing it.

Angular values defined at the surfaces separating the septal-lateral regions have to be extended to the whole anatomical site $\mathcal{M}_\theta$ to define b_θ. Since in this case $\mathcal{M}_\theta$ is given by the basal ring boundary, we independently solve the Laplacian for endocardium, epicardium, basal ring upper surface and SA lower plane with boundary conditions given by the intersection of the planes defining the septal and lateral regions with each of the 4 surfaces. The solutions to these Laplacians are used as boundary conditions in the second system of (2) to extend the angular coordinate to the whole volumetric mesh.

Elevation Coordinate. The elevation coordinate φ is defined in SA along the ventricular basal region and ranges from 0.65 at the lowest plane to 1 at the upper surface. These values are extended to $\mathcal{M}_\varphi$ given as before by the whole basal region boundary to define b_φ. To do so, we solve 2 Laplacian systems, one for the endocardium and another for the epicardium, with boundary conditions fixing their intersection with the basal ring to 1.0 and their intersection with the lower SA cut to 0.65. Finally, we propagate this elevation coordinate over the whole basal volume using these solutions to the Laplacian as boundary conditions in the 3rd system of (2).

3   Results

To illustrate the performance of the method, we have parameterized the ventricular basal region of 3 normal hearts from JHU canine cardiac database, labeled as DT080803, DT101703 and DT102403.

Figure 3 shows the 3 coordinate maps (r in 1st row, θ in 2nd row and φ in 3rd row) and the remeshing for the 3 cases in the last row. Remeshings show each coordinate isoline in a different color, red for r, green for θ and blue for φ. We observe that the propagation of each coordinate fixed at its specific anatomical site is smooth and homogeneous. This guarantees that the parametric map will be differentiable and will provide regular remeshings. The quality of the remeshing can be observed in the meshes of the last row, where we show the isolines of each coordinate map. It is worth noticing that their distribution over basal region is homogeneous in the 3 cases, which is a desirable property for a further use in cardiac models.

4   Discussion

The definition of reference frames, or unitary domains, that allow to compare different cardiac geometries in a meaningful way has several applications such as shape and function analysis or integration of data from different modalities. In this paper we have presented a method to obtain parameterizations of the left ventricle basal ring into a unitary domain. Moreover, with our method, we can go one step further and fix coordinate values in the unitary domain at anatomical features to force a more meaningful coordinate assignment.

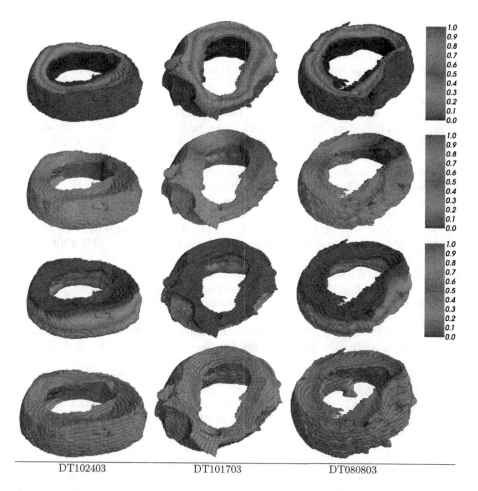

DT102403   DT101703   DT080803

Fig. 3. Results of constrained coordinate extension. Top row: radial coordinate r. Second row: angular coordinate θ. Third row: elevation coordinate φ. Bottom row: isolines over the volume for each coordinate by color $(red, green, blue) = (r, \theta, \varphi)$ (Color figure online)

In order to be able to compare different anatomies in the unitary domain, the definition of the anatomical landmarks to be set as interior boundary conditions plays a central role. Further analysis in this direction will be carried out. But the simplicity of the method and its robust mathematical background makes it a promising way to obtain a normalized anatomical space. On the other hand, other unitary domains, different from the unitary cube should be studied, in order to allow a clear definition of the apex central point and to take into account the right ventricle, specially the junction between its free wall and the septum.

References

1. Carapella, V., Bordas, R., Pathmanathan, P., et al.: Quantitative study of the effect of tissue microstructure on contraction in a computational model of rat left ventricle. PloS One **9**(4), e92792 (2014)
2. Casero, R., Burton, R.A.B., Quinn, T.A., Bollensdorff, C., Hales, P., Schneider, J.E., Kohl, P., Grau, V.: Towards high-resolution cardiac atlases: ventricular anatomy descriptors for a standardized reference frame. In: Camara, O., Pop, M., Rhode, K., Sermesant, M., Smith, N., Young, A. (eds.) STACOM 2010. LNCS, vol. 6364, pp. 75–84. Springer, Heidelberg (2010). doi:10.1007/978-3-642-15835-3_8
3. Desbrun, M., Meyer, M., Alliez, P.: Intrinsic parameterizations of surface meshes. Comput. Graph. Forum **21**, 209–218 (2002)
4. Evans, L.C.: Partial Differential Equations. American Mathematical Society, Providence (1998)
5. Garcia-Barnes, J., Gil, D., Badiella, L., et al.: A normalized framework for the design of feature spaces assessing the left ventricular function. TMI **29**(3), 733–745 (2010)
6. Gil, D., et al.: What a difference in biomechanics cardiac fiber makes. In: Camara, O., Mansi, T., Pop, M., Rhode, K., Sermesant, M., Young, A. (eds.) STACOM 2012. LNCS, vol. 7746, pp. 253–260. Springer, Heidelberg (2013). doi:10.1007/978-3-642-36961-2_29
7. Glocker, B., Sotiras, A., Komodakis, N., Paragios, N.: Deformable medical image registration: setting the state of the art with discrete methods*. Ann. Rev. Biomed. Eng. **13**, 219–244 (2011)
8. Gurgui, A., Gil, D., Marti, E.: Laplacian unitary domain for texture morphing. In: VISAPP (2015)
9. Helm, P., Beg, M.F., Miller, M.I., et al.: Measuring and mapping cardiac fiber and laminar architecture using diffusion tensor MR imaging. Ann. N. Y. Acad. Sci. **1047**, 296–307 (2005)
10. Karim, R., et al.: Surface flattening of the human left atrium and proof-of-concept clinical applications. Comput. Med. Imag. Graph **38**, 251–266 (2014)
11. Lamata, P., Niederer, S., Nordsletten, D., et al.: An accurate, fast and robust method to generate patient-specific cubic hermite meshes. Med. Image Anal. **15**(6), 801–813 (2011)
12. Lombaert, H., Grady, L., Pennec, X., Ayache, N., Cheriet, F.: Spectral log-demons: diffeomorphic image registration with very large deformations. IJCV **107**(3), 254–271 (2014)
13. Medrano-Gracia, P., Cowan, B.R., Suinesiaputra, A., et al.: Atlas-based anatomical modeling and analysis of heart disease. Drug Disc. Today Dis. Models **14**, 33–39 (2015)
14. Paun, B., Bijnens, B., Butakoff, C.: Subject independent reference frame for the left ventricular detailed cardiac anatomy. In: van Assen, H., Bovendeerd, P., Delhaas, T. (eds.) FIMH 2015. LNCS, vol. 9126, pp. 240–247. Springer, Heidelberg (2015). doi:10.1007/978-3-319-20309-6_28
15. Poveda, F., Marti, E., Andaluz, A., et al.: Helical structure of the cardiac ventricular anatomy assessed by diffusion tensor magnetic resonance imaging multiresolution tractography. Revista Española de Cardiología **66**(10), 782–790 (2013)
16. Soto-Iglesias, D., Butakoff, C., Andreu, D., et al.: Integration of electro-anatomical and imaging data of the left ventricle: an evaluation framework. Med. Image Anal. **32**, 131–144 (2016)

17. Vera, S., Ballester, M.A.G., Gil, D.: Anatomical parameterization for volumetric meshing of the liver. In: SPIE (2014)

18. Vera, S., González, M.A., Linguraru, M.G., Gil, D.: Optimal medial surface generation for anatomical volume representations. In: Yoshida, H., Hawkes, D., Vannier, M.W. (eds.) ABD-MICCAI 2012. LNCS, vol. 7601, pp. 265–273. Springer, Heidelberg (2012). doi:10.1007/978-3-642-33612-6_28

19. Young, A.A., Frangi, A.F.: Computational cardiac atlases: from patient to population and back. Exp. Physiol. **94**, 578–596 (2009)

Quasi-Conformal Technique for Integrating and Validating Myocardial Tissue Characterization in MRI with Ex-Vivo Human Histological Data

David Soto-Iglesias[1]([⊠]), Diego Penela[2], Xavier Planes[3], Veronika Zimmer[4], Juan Acosta[2], David Andreu[2], Gemma Piella[4], Rafael Sebastian[5], Damian Sancher-Quintana[6], Antonio Berruezo[2], and Oscar Camara[1]

[1] PhySense, DTIC, Universitat Pompeu Fabra, Barcelona, Spain
david.soto@upf.edu
[2] Cardiology Department, Arrhythmia Section,
Thorax Institute, Hospital Clinic, Barcelona, Spain
[3] GalgoMedical, Barcelona, Spain
[4] SIMBioSys, DTIC, Universitat Pompeu Fabra, Barcelona, Spain
[5] Computational Multi-Scale Physiology Lab,
Universitat de València, València, Spain
[6] Department of Anatomy and Cell Biology,
Universidad de Extremadura, Badajoz, Spain

Abstract. Ventricular tachycardia caused by a circuit of re-entry is one of the most critical arrhythmias. It is usually related with heterogeneous scar regions where slow velocity of conduction tissue is mixed with non-conductive tissue, creating pathways (CC) responsible for the tachycardia. Pre-operative DE-MRI can provide information on myocardial tissue viability and then improve therapy planning. However, the current DE-MRI resolution is not sufficient for identifying small CCs and therefore they have to be identified during the intervention, which requires considerable operator experience. In this work, we studied the relationship of histological data (with $10\,\mu m$ resolution), with in-vivo DE-MRI pixel intensities (PI) of one human heart. Integrating multi-modal data provided by different nature (in- vs. ex-vivo; 3D volume vs. 2D slices) is not straightforward and requires a robust integration pipeline. The main purpose of this work, is to develop a new technique for integrating histological information into the corresponding DE-MRI one. The proposed quasi-conformal mapping technique (QCM) integration were compared with state-of-the-art registration techniques (affine and non-rigid) on a benchmark of 418 synthetically generated datasets showing a more robust results. We used the QCM to quantitatively compare DE-MRI PI with the percentage of fibrosis extracted from histology. We show a positive correlation between the DE-MRI PI and the percentage of fibrosis extracted from histology ($r = 0.97$; $p < 0.0001$). Furthermore, we found a significant amount of viable tissue (up to 50%) in areas commonly defined as core zone in DE-MRI (PI level $> 60\%$ of the maximum intensity value).

© Springer International Publishing AG 2017
T. Mansi et al. (Eds.): STACOM 2016, LNCS 10124, pp. 172–181, 2017.
DOI: 10.1007/978-3-319-52718-5_19

Keywords: Registration · MRI · Cardiac arrhythmias · Histological data

1   Introduction

Ventricular tachycardia (VT) is one of the most critical arrhythmia, since it can lead to ventricular fibrillation and therefore to sudden cardiac death. Scar heterogeneous regions are composed by non-conductive tissue (core zone (CZ)) mixed with slow velocity of conduction tissue (border zone (BZ)) that can create a pathway (conduction channels, CC) responsible of the VT. The recommended treatment for VT's elimination (when the drugs failed) is to find pathophysio-logical electrograms (EGM) and eliminate them with radio frequency ablation (RFA). Most recently, the so called dechanelling technique proposed to ablate only the CC entrances reducing both the ablation area and the recurrences [1]. The ablation procedure is guided by a navigation system that fuse the electrical information integrated with 3D anatomy in an electro-anatomical map (EAM), which has been used for characterizing the tissue into healthy tissue (HT), BZ and CZ [2]. But, identifying all CC's during the procedure requires an expert operator and it is highly time-consuming. Pre-operative delayed-enhancement MRI (DE-MRI) can be used for classifying the myocardial tissue and there-fore identifying CC's and potential ablation targets. This classification is mainly based on pixel intensity (PI) thresholds [2]. However, the amount of CC's identi-fyed with DE-MRI and EAMs is different, as it was reported by [3], where they found a CCss match of 79.2% between both modalities. Histological information is close to be the gold standard for validating DE-MRI tissue classification. Cur-rent experimental studies have compared MRI and histological data on infarcted experimental swine models [4,5]. However, they only provide a partial histolog-ical analysis of some histological slices. Here, we propose to use high resolution histological data (a total of 80 histological slices with a resolution of $10\,\mu m$) of one ischemic patient for analyzing the relationship between in-vivo DE-MRI PI and the real scar configuration.

Registering multi-modal information acquired in different physical states, such as 3D in-vivo DE-MRI and 2D ex-vivo histological data is not straightfor-ward and requires an advanced integration pipeline. In [6] they reported that affine registration does not have to improve rigid-based registration results since the deformations rarely are only stretch or shear, instead they deform in more complex ways. Free-form deformation (FFD) based on splines has been sucess-fully used for non-rigid registration purpose [7]. However, no one has tested these techniques for registering imaging with histological data. In this paper, we intro-duced a new integration algorithm that successfully integrates histological and imaging data. We developed a synthetic histological dataset within which we can validate our method in comparison with affine and FFD non-rigid registra-tion algorithms. Applying our methodology to histological data we quantitatively relate each PI level presented in DE-MRI with the percentage of fibrosis observed in histology.

1) Original DE-MRI   2) DE-MRI Segmentation   3) Original histology   4) Histology mask registered   5) Fibrosis percentage

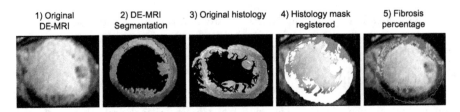

Fig. 1. One slice of Sect. 4 (S4) of the heart. (1) Original DE-MRI; (2) DE-MRI segmentation with 40% (green), 60% (red) and 70% (black) of maximum intensity value contours; (3) Original histological data; (4) High-resolution histological segmentation registered onto MRI; (5) Fibrosis percentage map. (Color figure online)

2 Clinical and Synthetic Data

2.1 Clinical Data

We analyze in-vivo DE-MRI and histological information of one ischemic patient with severe heart failure that went transplanted at Hospital Clinic de Barcelona.

MRI. The patient had a DE-MRI examination prior to the explantation, using a 3 T clinical scanner (Magnetom Trio, Siemens Healthcare). The 3D slab of images was acquired in the transaxial direction. Slice thickness was 1.4 mm, with no gap between slices. The field of view was set at $360\,mm^2$ and the matrix size was kept to 256×256 pixels in order to yield an isotropic spatial resolution of $1.4 \times 1.4 \times 1.4$ mm and getting a final resolution of $0.7 \times 0.7 \times 1.4$ mm.

Histology. After the heart extraction, a polymere (Vinyl Polysiloxane, HenrySchein) was introduced inside the heart for preserving the heart shape and preserved into formol, until sectioned. The complete heart was serially sectioned in the longitudinal apex-to-base direction into blocks of 1 cm thickness, resulting in 7 different blocks. Each block was divided into sections that fit on a 7.5×5 mm plate dimension but preserving the zone of interest (scar zone). Each section was embedded into paraffin wax and sectioned serially into slices of 10 microns thickness, with a rotation microtome (Microm HM340 E, Thermo Fisher Scientific, Walldorf, Germany). Every 20th section was stained with Masson trichrome relying in a mean of 20 slices per section. Finally, all the slices were digitalized with an Epson Perfection V600 Photo scanner, in keeping with previous studies [8]. Figure 1. illustrates one slice of mid-myocardium section (Sect. 4 of 7) together with the corresponding 2D MRI slice.

2.2 Generation of Synthetic Data

A set of synthetic data was generated to simulate MRI 2D slices (in short axis) and introducing some deformations to mimic the histological acquisition process.

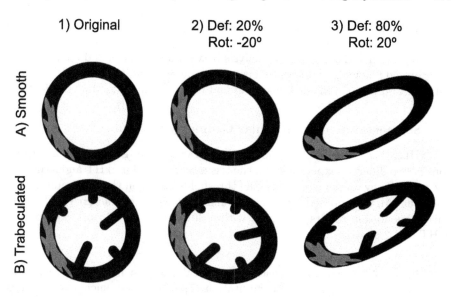

Fig. 2. Synthetic data: (A) Smooth model (B) Trabeculated model; (1) Model without deformations; (2) Model after 20% deformation and $-20°$ rotation; (3) Model after 80% deformation and 25° rotation.

Two different types of synthetic images were generated: (a) one with a smooth endocardium; and (b) another with a trabeculated endocardium. We simulated the myocardium as two concentric circles with a myocardium wall thickness of 4 cm. Additionally, we introduced a patch of fibrotic tissue on the septal wall, while trabecular structures were randomly generated including some cylinders in the endocardial wall, as can be seen in Fig. 2.

In order to simulate the effect of the heart extraction process, we applied a stretching in the antero-posterior direction and a dilation in the latero-septal one. We created the deformation matrix by modifying 8 control points (4 for the stretching and 4 for the dilatation) on the original image. We placed 2 control points at each image edge. To each control point, we applied 10 different levels of deformation, with a maximum deformation of 45°, which resulted in deformations from 0% to 100% with a resolution of 4.5°. Subsequently, we assumed that the effect of the slicing process in histology could be simulated as a set of image rotations from $-45°$ to 45°. Finally, for simulating intra-section displacements, we randomly applied translations in the x and y axes with a maximum of ± 2.5 cm. All these transformations resulted in a dataset composed of 418 different synthetic images with different levels of deformations. Figure 2. depicts two examples with different percentages of rotational angles and deformations.

3   Methods

The integration and quantitative analysis between histological and imaging data is performed following 3 different steps: (1) tissue segmentation (in DE-MRI and histological data); (2) 2D disk mapping and registration; and (3) quantification.

3.1   Segmentation of Ventricular Geometry and Substrate

DE-MRI. The LV geometry is manually extracted from DE-MRI by a consensious of two different experts. Then, the tissue is classified into HT and scar zone (BZ and CZ) by applying the baseline thresholds based on the maximum intensity value (MIV) proposed by [2] and usually applied to characterize CCs [1,3]. This segmentation results in a mask with 3 different values: 0 as background, 1 as HT and 2 as scar.

Histology. We down-sample each histological 2D slice from $7.8 \times 7.6 \,\mu m$ to $34 \times 28 \,\mu m$ for improving the computational performance, such resolution is acceptable compared with the DE-MRI one ($70 \times 70 \,\mu m$). Then, we segment each image into HT (viable myocardium, in red) and fibrosis (collagen and fat, in green and white respectively), as can be seen on Fig. 1. We use each LAB color channel for classifying the myocardium into: background (L channel), HT (B channel) and fibrosis (A channel). We compute a weighted final mask according to the DE-MRI segmentation one. Finally, we manually eliminate the right ventricle and resize the high-resolution (HR) histological mask to the MRI resolution prior to the registration.

3.2   Registration Techniques

Each 2D histological slice is automatically associated with its correspondent DE-MRI one following the sectioning order. For that purpose, we use three different approaches: (i) An affine 2D registration [6]; (ii) A FFD non-rigid registration [7] applied after the affine; and (iii) A new method based on a quasi-conformal mapping (QCM), in concordance with previous studies [9].

Quasi-conformal Mapping (QCM) on Imaging Data. We extend the QCM introduced by previoius studies to also integrate multi-modal images [9]. QCM requires a set of vertices and their connectivity, so we transform each 2D image to the mesh domain, meaning a set of vertices and their connectivity instead of pixels. We consider each pixel inside the myocardium as a vertex of the mesh, subsequently we applied a Delaunay triangulation for computing their connectivity. The myocardium in short axis has the shape of a donut and it is homeomorphic to a disk. This homeomorphism can be computed by requiring that every vertex coordinate of the triangulation has a vanishing conformal Laplacian. By mapping both DE-MRI and histological 2D slices on the same disk we can establish a piecewise linear homeomorphism between the two surfaces. In order to have an unique solution to the laplacian equation we just need to select one landmark. We choose one located on the middle of the septum (MS) and it is mapped to the $[-1, 0]$ XY coordinate system. Additionally, we automatically select another landmark in the gravity center of the mesh that will be mapped on the center of the disk. Once we know the mapping transformation from DE-MRI to the disk and the one from histology to the disk, we can consider them as two different triangulations of the same disk. Based on barycentric coordinates, we can associate scalars information from histology to DE-MRI vertices. Furthermore, we perform a rigid registration on the disk domain for minimizing the MS dependence. We apply a spin to the histological disk for maximizing the overlap with the DE-MRI one. At this point, applying the DE-MRI inverse mapping will result in the histological information mapped on the DE-MRI coordinate system. The whole mapping process is also applied to the HR histological mesh.

3.3   Quantification

Having both DE-MRI and HR histology on the same system of coordinates we can establish relationship between their vertices. First, we associate each HR histological vertex to the closest DE-MRI one. Then, for each DE-MRI vertex we compute the percentage of HR vertices classified as fibrosis (fibrosis map) and the ones classified as HT (tissue map). At this point, for each DE-MRI pixel intensity level we compute the mean percentage of fibrosis and viable tissue.

4   Results

Registration Accuracy. The registration accuracy was evaluated by computing the multi-fractional generalized Tanimoto coefficient (TC_{MF}) [10] on the synthetic dataset. Figure 3 depicts the TC_{MF} (mean $\pm$ standard deviation) achieved by each registration technique for different applied deformations. A Wilcoxon signed-rank test was applied to estimate the significance of differences between the QCM and the other alternatives, a p-value < 0.05 indicates statistically significant differences. The overall mean TC_{MF} was of: 0.80 ± 0.15 for affine, 0.93 ± 0.08 for FFD and 0.93 ± 0.04 for QCM. The QCM method performed better than the affine method for both models and independently of the amount of deformation applied. However, registration accuracy provided by all strategies depended on the amount of deformation introduced. For the smooth model, accuracy results were similar for all registration methods up to 50 % of the maximum deformation, even if QCM was slightly better. For larger deformations ($>70\%$), the affine registration did not work at the same level of the FFD and QCM methods, which were not significantly different. In general, the overlap values were lower with the trabeculated than with the smooth model. The trabeculated model showed that an affine transformation was not enough to cope with this type of differences between the images to register. Interestingly, QCM performed slightly better than FFD for deformations up to 40% of the maximum value, while the opposite behavior was found for larger deformations.

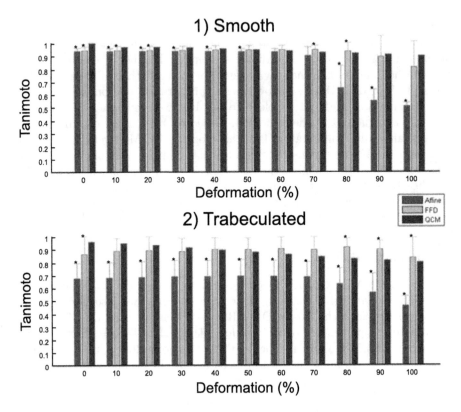

Fig. 3. Mean TC_{MF} overlap per amount of deformation (from 0% to 100%) for: (1) Smooth model and (2) Trabeculated model; Red: Affine; Green: Affine + FFD; Blue: QCM. * Represent statistically differences between each method result and QCM. (Color figure online)

Figure 4 depicts the registration results obtained on the synthetic data shown in Fig. 2, illustrating how QCM could correctly locate the main features of interest (e.g. scar zone or trabeculae) independently of the imposed amount of deformation. Nevertheless, the QCM did not correctly recover myocardial thickness in some spatial locations with high deformations.

DE-MRI vs. Histological Quantification. Figure 1 depicts the results of the HR histology QCM registration together with the percentage of fibrosis for one slice of the mid-myocardium, Sect. 4 (S4). After the registration, we performed a quantification of the percentage of fibrosis at each pixel intensity level, the results for S4 and for overall sections are illustrated on Fig. 5. The two vertical lines correspond to the 40% and 60% thresholds generally used to characterize the myocardium [2]. One can observe significant amount of viable tissue (up to 50%) at zones previously considered as CZ (red area on Fig. 5). The percentage of

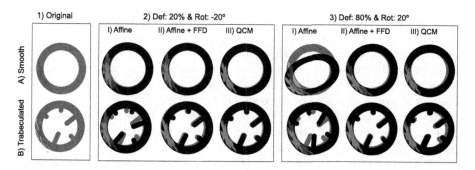

Fig. 4. Registration results with: (i) Affine; (ii) Affine + FFD; and (iii) QCM for two different synthetic models. (1) Both models: (A) Smooth and (B) Trabeculated; (2) Deformation of 20% and rotation of $-20°$; and (3) Deformation of 80% with rotation of $20°$.

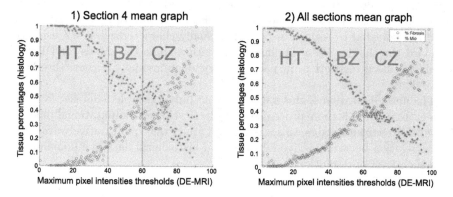

Fig. 5. 2D graph for all sections; x axis: percentage of the maximum intensity value; y axis: percentage of fibrosis (blue circles) and viable tissue (red stars). Healthy tissue (HT) is considered as pixel intensity (PI) level lower than 40%, border zone (BZ) as PI levels between 40% and 60% and core zone (CZ) as PI levels higher than 60%; purple, green and red colors represent the HT, BZ and CZ zones respectively. (Color figure online)

fibrosis is positively correlated with the PI level 0.97 p-value < 0.0001 for overall sections.

5   Discussion and Conclusions

The main objective of this paper was to present a quantitative comparison of scar characterizations derived from corresponding histological and in-vivo DE-MRI data on an human heart. The developed computational pipeline improved the results on synthetic data comparing to other commonly applied methods such as affine and FFD for amounts of deformations in the range of the studied data (Fig. 4). However, for larger deformations a combined registration approach such as affine+FFD seemed to also provide good registration accuracy, even if presenting a larger variance than when using QCM. This high variance pointed out that applying a non-rigid registration without regularization constraints can substantially deform small structures such as scar or trabecular regions, producing aberrant results. These aberrations are minimized with QCM since it preserves the original shape of the registered surfaces.

The developed computational pipeline successfully integrated both types of multi-modal information into the same reference system, reconstructing the multi-slice 2D histological ex-vivo data into the 3D LV geometry defined by the DE-MRI in-vivo data. In this way, a point-by-point comparison between relevant indices from both modalities, such as percentage of fibrotic tissue and PI from histology and DE-MRI, respectively, was possible. The quantitative multi-modal scar analysis revealed two main findings: (i) DE-MRI PI presents a positive correlation with the percentage of fibrosis presented on histological data (0.97 p-value < 0.0001 for overall sections) and therefore it can be used for tissue classification purposes; and (ii) a significant amount of viable tissue (up to 30%) is associated to regions in DE-MRI usually characterized as CZ using the standard thresholds. These findings suggest that these thresholds for DE-MRI should be more restrictive, in particular for defining the CZ (new thresholds above 60%).

The main limitation of this study was that only a complete dataset from one patient was available to be processed with the developed computational pipeline. However, to our knowledge, this was the first study that quantitatively evaluated the correlation between in-vivo DE-MRI and histological data in a human heart with such level of resolution.

References

1. Berruezo, A., Fernández-Armenta, J., Andreu, D., Penela, D., Herczku, C., Evertz, R., Cipolletta, L., Acosta, J., Borràs, R., Arbelo, E., et al.: Scar dechanneling: a new method for scar-related left ventricular tachycardia substrate ablation. Circ. Arrhythmia Electrophysiol. CIRCEP-114 (2015)
2. Andreu, D., Berruezo, A., Ortiz-Pérez, J., Silva, E., Mont, L., Borràs, R., de Caralt, T., Perea, R., Fernández-Armenta, J., Zeljko, H., Brugada, J.: Integration of 3D electroanatomic maps and magnetic resonance scar characterization into the navigation system to guide ventricular tachycardia ablation. Circ. Arrhythmia Electrophysiol. 4(5), 674–683 (2011)
3. Andreu, D., Ortiz-Pérez, J.T., Fernández-Armenta, J., Guiu, E., Acosta, J., Prat-González, S., De Caralt, T.M., Perea, R.J., Garrido, C., Mont, L., et al.: 3d delayed-enhanced magnetic resonance sequences improve conducting channel delineation prior to ventricular tachycardia ablation. Europace 17(6), 938–945 (2015)
4. Tschabrunn, C.M., Roujol, S., Nezafat, R., Faulkner-Jones, B., Buxton, A.E., Josephson, M.E., Anter, E.: A swine model of infarct-related reentrant ventricular tachycardia: electroanatomic, magnetic resonance, and histopathological characterization. Heart Rhythm 13(1), 262–273 (2016)

5. Pop, M., Ghugre, N., Ramanan, V., Morikawa, L., Stanisz, G., Dick, A., Wright, G.: Quantification of fibrosis in infarcted swine hearts by ex vivo late gadolinium-enhancement and diffusion-weighted mri methods. Phys. Med. Biol. **58**(15), 5009 (2013)
6. Hill, D.L., Batchelor, P.G., Holden, M., Hawkes, D.J.: Medical image registration. Phys. Med. Biol. **46**(3), R1 (2001)
7. Rueckert, D., Somoda, I., Hayes, C., Hill, D., Leach, M., Hawkes, D.: Nonrigid registration using free-form deformations: applications to breast MR images. IEEE Trans. Med. Imaging **18**(8), 712–721 (1999)
8. Keith, A., Flack, M.: The form and nature of the muscular connections between the primary divisions of the vertebrate heart. J. Anat. Physiol. **41**(Pt. 3), 172 (1907)
9. Soto-Iglesias, D., Butakoff, C., Andreu, D., Fernández-Armenta, J., Berruezo, A., Camara, O.: Integration of electro-anatomical and imaging data of the left ventricle: an evaluation framework. Med. Image Anal. **32**, 131–144 (2016)
10. Crum, W., Camara, O., Hill, D.: Generalized overlap measures for evaluation and validation in medical image analysis. IEEE Trans. Med. Imaging **25**(11), 1451–1461 (2006)

Myocardial Scar Quantification Using SLIC Supervoxels - Parcellation Based on Tissue Characteristic Strains

Iulia A. Popescu[1(✉)], Benjamin Irving[1], Alessandra Borlotti[2],
Erica Dall'Armellina[2], and Vicente Grau[1]

[1] Department of Engineering Science, Institute of Biomedical Engineering,
University of Oxford, Oxford, UK
iulia.popescu@eng.ox.ac.uk
[2] Department of Cardiovascular Medicine, Acute Vascular Imaging Centre (AVIC),
University of Oxford, Oxford, UK

Abstract. Abnormal myocardial motion occurs in many cardiac pathologies, though in different ways, depending on the disease, some of which can result in negative clinical outcomes. Therefore, a better understanding of the contractile capability of the tissue is crucial in providing an improved and patient-specific clinical outcome [4]. Cardiovascular Magnetic Resonance Imaging (CMR) is considered the gold standard for the assessment of cardiac function and has the potential to also be used for routine tissue strain analysis because of its high availability in clinical practice. In this study we estimate the local strain in myocardial tissue over a cardiac cycle using cine MRI imaging to perform the analysis. To quantify the tissue displacement, we use the diffeomorphic demons registration algorithm [15] in a multi-step 3D registration, for the minimization of cumulative errors propagation. Using the displacement gradient of the deformation, individual voxel strain curves are computed. We present a novel method for parcellating the myocardium into regions based on the strain behaviour of clusters of voxels. We define the supervoxels using the Simple Linear Iterative Clustering (SLIC) algorithm [1] inside a predefined mask. The results are consistent with late gadolinium enhancement scar identification.

1 Introduction

Accurate quantification of myocardial contraction and relaxation is fundamental for a comprehensive analysis of cardiac health. One of the earliest methods for tracking myocardial motion is based on the implantation of radiopaque fiducial markers, however due to its invasive nature, this method was never applicable in clinical practice. Echocardiography, either using Tissue Doppler or speckle tracking, can be used to estimate myocardial motion and strain. However, the angular dependence of tissue velocity measurements, the low spatial resolution of the images, as well as the difficulty to image both ventricles at the same time, significantly limit its usability.

© Springer International Publishing AG 2017
T. Mansi et al. (Eds.): STACOM 2016, LNCS 10124, pp. 182–190, 2017.
DOI: 10.1007/978-3-319-52718-5_20

Tagged MRI is generally accepted as the current gold standard for quantification of myocardial motion in the clinical setting. The method uses spin tagging prepulses to produce a magnetized rigid grid on the image [2], and subsequently the grid deformation is tracked over a cardiac cycle. However, one of the main limitations of the method is that is not used in routine clinical practice, and therefore restricted to research hospitals. Furthermore the acquisition requires significant more time in the scanner compared to cine MRI.

Cine MRI is considered the gold standard in clinical practice for tissue characterisation. However, its use for the quantification of tissue deformation and strain has also been explored. Previous methods include tissue tracking using diffeomorphic registration algorithms with a superimposed incompressibility criteria for volume preservation [10], or with physical constrains such as divergence free deformations and myocardium elasticity modelling [11] to extract the strain curves. More recently, Bai et al. [3] have investigated the division of left ventricle based on tissue displacements using a hierarchical clustering method, where the number of clusters were set to be equivalent to the number of segments in the 17 segments model. The method proposed in this paper differs from [3] in that we are not aiming to divide the myocardium into segments, but to identify the region/regions that have been affected by pathology. While the concept of local division, or parcellation, is not new to biomedical image analysis, being extensively used brain applications, it is only recently that has been used in cardiac applications.

The standard clinical method for the quantification of scarred tissue - post myocardial infarction, is late gadolinium enhancement (LGE). The concept is based on the delayed wash-in and wash-out effect in tissue where the space between cells is significantly higher than normal tissue - e.g. in the case of post myocardial infarction scar. While LGE provides critical information for patient diagnosis and management, its combination with motion analysis provides a more complete picture of structure-function relationship in cardiac disease. More recently, imaging methods for scar quantification have been proposed based on motion patterns [12] and quantification of the myocardial deformation [5], where the aim is to replace the need to use contrast enhancement agents, like in the case of conventional LGE.

Cardiac strain can be used to summarise tissue deformation and is thus directly related to structural properties of the tissue. Spottiswoode et al. [13] use cine DENSE MRI to compute the radial and circumferential strains. Mansi et al. [11] use Physically Constrained Diffeomorphic Demons to estimate the circumferential and radial strains from cine MRI.

In this work we present **a novel method for the quantification of myocardial strain from cine MRI sequences using individual voxel strain curves**, grouped using a supervoxel algorithm. Our main contribution is the development of a parcellation method for the division of the left ventricle into regions based on tissue characteristic radial strain, which has the potential of improving tissue strain analysis. For this purpose we also present a method for spatial tracking of discrete material points (voxels) of the myocardium during myocardial motion, and subsequently build strain curves of the tracked voxels over a cardiac cycle. We provide initial validation by comparing results with LGE images.

2   Materials

The data set used for this publication is part of the OxAMI (Oxford Acute Myocardial Infarction) clinical study, which was provided by the University of Oxford Centre for Clinical Magnetic Resonance Research at the John Radcliffe Hospital, Oxford. The images were acquired on a 3.0T Siemens TIM-Trio whole-body MRI scanner, using steady-state free precession (SSFP) for cine imaging, and were gated to the vector ECG. The LGE images were acquired in the same session. The dataset used for this publication consist of nine cases, where each of cases has the following image characteristics: 25 time frames per slice, a voxel size of $1.56 \times 1.56\,mm^2$ and a slice thickness of 8 mm.

The segmentation of the left ventricle (LV) was done manually by an expert cardiologist, where for each time frames the endocardium and epicardium is segmented using the (cmr^{42}) software (Circle Cardiovascular Imaging, Calgary, Alberta, Canada).

3   Methods

3.1   Data Preprocessing

We reconstruct the 4D volume (3D + time), from 2D slices, using trilinear interpolation in the z direction, in order to ensure voxel isotropy. The volume generated has isotropic voxel size of $1.56 \times 1.56 \times 1.56\,mm^3$.

3.2   Diffeomorphic Log Demons Image Registration Algorithm

Diffeomorphic Demons registration algorithm is a non-parametric, non-rigid, image registration algorithm. The algorithm consists of two terms: a similarity criteria, and a regularisation term (a Gaussian smoothing filter in this case). The displacement of each voxel is calculated using the intensity similarities between a static (reference) and a moving image. For this paper we use an implementation developed by Dirk-Jan Kroon [9]. Our method applies this algorithm within a multiple step registration process, designed to minimise accumulation of errors. The final motion field is computed as follows: **First pass:** (a) Consecutive frames are aligned to each other in an descending order; (b) Pre-aligned frames are aligned to the reference frame (last); **Second pass:** (a) Consecutive frames are aligned to each other in an ascending order; (b) Pre-aligned frames are aligned to the reference frame (first). Both deformation fields are then combined, using a weighting function, according to the distance between each frame and the reference frame. While an incompressible version, iLog Demons, is available, the lack of an open-source implementation and the good results obtained by Log Demons made us choose the latter.

3.3   Strain Estimation

The gradient of the deformation quantifies the change in shape of infinitesimal line elements in a solid body. To explain the concept let us take a straight, infinitely small line, d_x, on an undeformed configuration of a solid, and deform the volume. Now let us call the deformed line, d_y. The infinitesimal segments d_x and d_y are related by: $d_y = F{\cdot}d_x$, where F represents the gradient of the deformation matrix. To quantify the contractile function of the tissue, we compute the 3D Lagrangian strain tensor E. Here $E = 1/2(F^T F - I)$, with I representing the identity matrix.

The 3D Lagrangian strain tensor quantifies the changes in shape of a piece of tissue with respect to its original configuration. The analysis of the Lagrangian strain tensor provides a direct estimation of the magnitude of the deformation through six indices: 3 normal strains: radial, circumferential, and longitudinal and 3 pairs of shear strains. In this work we use the radial strain. The radial strain was chosen to serve as feature for proof of concept of dividing the LV into sections based on local strain patterns.

3.4   Left Ventricle Parcellation - SLIC Supervoxels

Simple Linear Iterative Clustering (SLIC) is a segmentation algorithm that divides an image into small clusters of pixels, called superpixels, by using local k-means clustering - defining a distance metric weighted between the pixel intensity and spatial similarity [1]. Because the superpixel/supervoxel segmentation is a method for dividing an image into a set of regions, based on local similarity, in our case, this approach can provide a more natural set of subregions for analysis. In conventional SLIC, k initial cluster centres are sampled on a rectangular grid, spaced $S = \sqrt{N/k}$ apart [1], where N is the number of pixels/voxels. In this work a 3D + time adaptation of the SLIC algorithm is used to generate the supervoxels [7]. The source code is available at (URL: https://github.com/ benjaminirving/perfusion-slic) to facilitate reimplementation. The key novelty is that we use shape characteristics of the strain curves to define each supervoxel region.

The main difference of our method with respect to conventional SLIC relies in the use of strain curves instead of image intensities. PCA modes of variation for dimensionality reduction [8] was used instead of all the available time points, in order to remove as much noise as possible from the strain curves. PCA is first applied to strain curves calculated for each voxel corresponding to myocardial tissue. The first three modes of variation from PCA are selected, and their values used to generate the supervoxels. Voxels are assigned to the nearest cluster centre using k-means clustering, with a 2S × 2S × 2S distance of each cluster, with a modified distance metric to include a feature distance term, using principal component analysis to extract these features [7]. An additional adaptation is that the supervoxalisation is only performed within the mask. This is done by placing equidistant seed points within the mask to initialise the SLIC using a distance transform derived method [6].

A supervoxel based step was used for a number of reasons, first the spatial regularisation reduces noise in the images and allows more robust features from each region, second, it provides meaningful regions for visual assessment, and finally it reduces the computational complexity of the analysis.

3.5 Dividing the Tissue According to Similar Patterns in Radial Strain Curves

Once the supervoxels have been calculated, we use them to obtain a division of the left ventricle into regions based on local tissue characteristic strains, as an alternative to the standard division into the AHA 17-segment model.

4   Results

For this study we used a set of nine myocardial infarction patients. The late gadolinium enhancement for scarred tissue images (Fig. 1(a) and (b)) were used to visually estimate the position and dimension of the scarred tissue. The corresponding slices, cine MRI (Fig. 1(c) and (d)) were the only ones used to compute the radial strain in the left ventricle. Both cine and LGE images were acquired in the same visit, typically 24 h after myocardial infarction patient was presented at the emergency care unit.

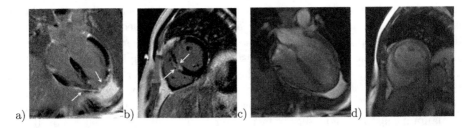

Fig. 1. Late gadolinium enhancement for myocardial infarction patient, case1 (a) and (b) and cine MRI matching slices for the same case, (c) and (d). One mention is that the LGE images are for only one time point, beginning of systolic phase.

From the 4D registered volume we extracted the displacement curves over a cardiac cycle, as explained in Sect. 3.2. Subsequently the LV mask is applied, and the supervoxels are generated inside the mask using as a feature the voxel individual strain curves. A 3D representation of the supervoxels distribution, as well as the three clusters build using tissue characteristic radial strain, can be seen in Fig. 2, for Case I (a) and Case IV (b). We use k-means clustering to separate the labeled supervoxels into three classes in the attempt to have a class for each of the following possibility of tissue being healthy, damaged, or affected but viable. However, this being only preliminary work, validation is needed in order to assign names to classes.

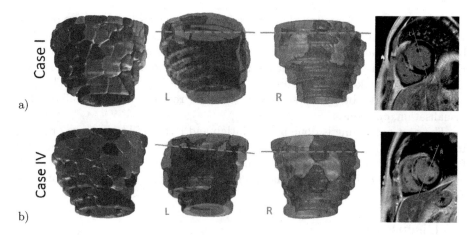

Fig. 2. Case I(a) and Case IV(b): From left to right: Left ventricle supervoxels generated using PCA three modes of variation on individual strain curves. Tissue clustered into three clusters using k-means, septal view (L = left). Tissue clustered into three clusters using k-means, lateral view (R = right). Corresponding LGE image.

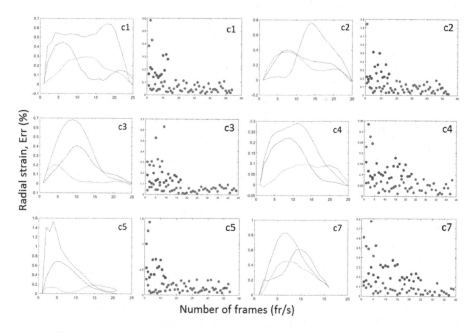

Fig. 3. Six cases: For each case, left to right: Mean strain curves for each cluster. K-means clustering into three labels according to peak value of mean strain curve for each supervoxel (the x axis is just to include it to distribute the data for visualisation purposes).

For Case 1 (c1), we found that the radial strain curves have a range of peak values between 10% and 60% as shown in Fig. 3. c1, where the lower value is believed to be pathology. Case 6 was excluded due to bad slice misalignment. For six of the cases a figure that summarises the mean strain curves for each cluster, as well as k-means clusters for each case can be seen in Fig. 3. The rest of three cases are not presented purely for space reasons, but are available for visualisation, on request.

The post-processing is done using Matlab and Python. The average processing times using a Intel i7, 16 GB (RAM) and 64-bit Windows operating system, for 25 volumes of a typical dataset are: complete cardiac cycle displacement curves - aprox 1 h; complete cardiac cycle strains computation per 25 volumes - aprox 134 s.

5   Discussion

Cine MRI is the most commonly used MRI imaging sequence in cardiac MRI imaging. Although currently used for the assessment of the global heart function and anatomy, it presents a great potential in the assessment of cardiac tissue structural changes. One of the advantages over techniques like tagged MRI, is the general availability, limited need for user interaction as well as the reduction of study time. However, low resolution in the z direction and limited texture analysis inside the myocardium, could potentially become limitations in using the cine MRI sequence for the computation of the strains.

We argue that while the 17 segments AHA model is very useful for the anatomical localisation of the infarction, this approach can introduce errors by not taking into consideration features like time to peak or peak strain value for individual voxels, or averaging curves with different peak times into a low peak strain curve, which might or might not be 'signaled' by the total average of the segment. Using a parcellation approach, like 3D modified SLIC, gives us the possibility to investigate individual voxels behaviour and subsequently group them according to similar motion patterns.

For this work we used only the radial strain, however, in the future we consider introducing both radial and circumferential, as well as longitudinal strain in the classifier to generate the supervoxels. The LV was chosen due to relatively easy segmentation compared to the right ventricle (RV), however, we consider extending the method to the RV in the future.

This work has potential to become a semi-automated tool, where clinicians could interact with the regions of supervoxels.

Strain calculation methods previously reported in the literature do not always agree on maximum peak strain. However, they report similar order of magnitude strains, with consistent strain curves shape morphology across methods. Maximum peak strain can vary depending on the registration algorithm used, whether the algorithm has a regularisation term or not, as explained in [14]. Registration algorithms that have no regularisation term tend to show higher maximum peak strain values, while registration algorithms that have a regularisation term tend to underestimate the radial strain in particular.

In future, there is potential for considering more features to characterise the strain curves. Once we've acquired clinical delineations of the infarcted regions we can extend this approach to supervised learning, however there is uncertainty in the clinical delineation in LGE, therefore, region-base cine MRI analysis offers an alternative. Also, a comparison of our method with other existing methods for scar quantification, will be considered.

K-means clustering represents a limitation at the moment, due to its tendency to always group into a predefined number of clusters. We plan to evaluate supervised learning methods in the future.

Acknowledgements. This research is supported by the RCUK Digital Economy Programme grant number EP/G036861/1, Oxford Centre for Doctoral Training in Healthcare Innovation. ED acknowledges the BHF intermediate clinical research fellow grant (FS/13/71/30378) and the NIHR BRC. VG is supported by a BBSRC grant (BB/I012117/1), an EPSRC grant (EP/J013250/1) and by BHF New Horizon Grant NH/13/30238.

References

1. Achanta, R., Shaji, A., Smith, K., Lucchi, A., Fua, P., Süsstrunk, S.: SLIC superpixels compared to state-of-the-art superpixel methods. IEEE Trans. Pattern Anal. Mach. Intell. **34**(11), 2274–2281 (2012)
2. Axel, L., Montillo, A., Kim, D.: Tagged magnetic resonance imaging of the heart a survey. Med. Image Anal. **9**, 376–393 (2005)
3. Bai, W., Peressutti, D., Parisot, S., Oktay, O., Rajchl, M., O'Regan, D., Cook, S., King, A., Rueckert, D.: Beyond the AHA 17-segment model: motion-driven parcellation of the left ventricle. In: Camara, O., Mansi, T., Pop, M., Rhode, K., Sermesant, M., Young, A. (eds.) STACOM 2015. LNCS, vol. 9534, pp. 13–20. Springer, Heidelberg (2016). doi:10.1007/978-3-319-28712-6_2
4. Dall'Armellina, E., Choudhury, R.P.: The role of cardiovascular magnetic resonance in patients with acute coronary syndromes. Progr. Cardiovasc. Dis. **54**(3), 230–239 (2011)
5. Duchateau, N., Sermesant, M.: Prediction of infarct localization from myocardial deformation. In: Camara, O., Mansi, T., Pop, M., Rhode, K., Sermesant, M., Young, A. (eds.) STACOM 2015. LNCS, vol. 9534, pp. 51–59. Springer, Heidelberg (2016). doi:10.1007/978-3-319-28712-6_6
6. Irving, B.: SLIC in a defined mask with applications to medical imaging, pp. 1–5 (2016). http://arxiv.org/abs/1606.09518
7. Irving, B., Franklin, J.M., Papiez, B.W., Anderson, E.M., Sharma, R.A., Gleeson, F.V., Brady, S.M., Schnabel, J.A.: Pieces-of-parts for supervoxel segmentation with global context: application to DCE-MRI tumour delineation. Med. Image Anal. **32**, 69–83 (2016)
8. Irving, B.J., Goussard, P., Andronikou, S., Gie, R., Douglas, T.S., Todd-Pokropek, A., Taylor, P.: Computer assisted detection of abnormal airway variation in CT scans related to paediatric tuberculosis. Med. Image Anal. **18**(7), 963–976 (2014)
9. Kroon, D.J., Slump, C.H.: MRI modalitiy transformation in demon registration. In: Proceedings of the Sixth IEEE International Conference on Symposium on Biomedical Imaging: From Nano to Macro, ISBI 2009, pp. 963–966. IEEE Press, Piscataway (2009)

10. Mansi, T., Pennec, X., Sermesant, M., Delingette, H., Ayache, N.: ILogDemons: a demons-based registration algorithm for tracking incompressible elastic biological tissues. Int. J. Comput. Vis. **92**(1), 92–111 (2011)
11. Mansi, T., Peyrat, J.-M., Sermesant, M., Delingette, H., Blanc, J., Boudjemline, Y., Ayache, N.: Physically-constrained diffeomorphic demons for the estimation of 3D myocardium strain from cine-MRI. In: Ayache, N., Delingette, H., Sermesant, M. (eds.) FIMH 2009. LNCS, vol. 5528, pp. 201–210. Springer, Heidelberg (2009). doi:10.1007/978-3-642-01932-6_22
12. Peressutti, D., Bai, W., Shi, W., Tobon-Gomez, C., Jackson, T., Sohal, M., Rinaldi, A., Rueckert, D., King, A.: Towards left ventricular scar localisation using local motion descriptors. In: Camara, O., Mansi, T., Pop, M., Rhode, K., Sermesant, M., Young, A. (eds.) STACOM 2015. LNCS, vol. 9534, pp. 30–39. Springer, Heidelberg (2016). doi:10.1007/978-3-319-28712-6_4
13. Spottiswoode, B.S., Zhong, X., Hess, A.T., Kramer, C.M., Meintjes, E.M., Mayosi, B.M., Epstein, F.H.: Tracking myocardial motion from cine DENSE images using spatiotemporal phase unwrapping and temporal fitting. IEEE Trans. Med. Imaging **26**(1), 15–30 (2007)
14. Tobon-Gomez, C., et al.: Benchmarking framework for myocardial tracking and deformation algorithms: an open access database. Med. Image Anal. **17**(6), 632–648 (2013)
15. Vercauteren, T., Pennec, X., Perchant, A., Ayache, N.: Diffeomorphic demons: efficient non-parametric image registration. NeuroImage **45**(Suppl. 1), S61–S72 (2009)

SLAWT (Segmentation of Left Atrial Wall Thickness) Challenge Papers

Segmentation Challenge on the Quantification of Left Atrial Wall Thickness

Rashed Karim[1]([✉]), Marta Varela[1], Pranav Bhagirath[3], Ross Morgan[1],
Jonathan M. Behar[1,2], R. James Housden[1], Ronak Rajani[2], Oleg Aslanidi[1],
and Kawal S. Rhode[1]

[1] Division of Imaging Sciences and Biomedical Engineering,
King's College London, London, UK
rashed.karim@kcl.ac.uk

[2] Department of Cardiology, Guy's and St. Thomas' NHS Foundation Trust,
London, UK

[3] Haga Teaching Hospital, The Hague, The Netherlands

Abstract. This paper presents an image database for the Left Atrial Wall Thickness Quantification challenge at the MICCAI STACOM 2016 workshop along with some preliminary results. The image database consists of both CT ($n = 10$) and MRI ($n = 10$) datasets. Expert delineations from two observers were obtained for each image in the CT set and a single-observer segmentation was obtained for each image in the MRI set included in this study. Computer algorithms for segmentation of wall thickness from three research groups contributed to this challenge. The algorithms were evaluated on the basis of wall thickness measurements obtained from the segmentation masks.

Keywords: Image segmentation · Left atrium · CT · Angiography · MRI · Image quantification

1 Introduction

Atrial fibrillation (AF) is the most common cardiac arrhythmia causing chaotic contraction of the atrium. AF becomes more prevalent with age [1], is frequently associated with atrial remodelling and fibrosis, and causes loss of atrial muscle mass, the severity of which reflects the duration of preexisting AF. Pulmonary vein isolation is often the first procedure performed in patients referred for catheter ablation of AF. The left atrium (LA) is known to undergo changes in structural and electrical behaviour with conditions that predispose AF [2]. Until recently, structural and electrical remodelling in the LA was not very well understood. Success of AF is now highly dependent upon the ability to create fully extent or *transmural* lesions within the LA wall.

The LA wall is a thin structure. Assessment of the LA has been restricted because of its size and blood flow. Measurement of the size of its wall has not been possible *in-vivo* until recently. At first, echocardiography was the only

T. Mansi et al. (Eds.): STACOM 2016, LNCS 10124, pp. 193–200, 2017.
DOI: 10.1007/978-3-319-52718-5_21

widely available tool for cardiac structural assessment, but it was not well suited because of its low spatial resolution. Transesophageal Echocardiography (TEE) provided higher spatial resolution and has been used to measure increases in wall thickness [3]. The availability of high-resolution imaging technology in CT and Cardiac Magnetic Resonance (CMR) has provided an accurate means of measuring its thickness. State-of-the-art image processing algorithms are also now becoming readily available as open source.

Due to the challenging nature of the problem of wall thickness segmentation and quantification, the Left Atrial Wall Thickness Quantification challenge was put forward publicly and three image processing research groups participated. This work aims to present some preliminary results.

2   Methods

2.1   Imaging Data

The image database consisted of CT ($n = 10$) and MRI ($n = 10$) datasets from separate groups of patients. The images were all obtained from a single centre. The CT datasets were obtained from coronary CT angiography scans, with an intravenous contrast agent injection. The scans were ECG-gated and acquired in a single breath hold. The images were reconstructed to a 0.8 to 1 mm slice thickness, with a 0.4 mm slice increment and a 250 mm field of view. The image matrix was kept at a 512×512 matrix, constructed with a sharp reconstruction kernel.

The MRI datasets were acquired with respiratory gating using a pencil-beam navigator and the average scan time was about 12 min. Cardiac triggering ensured that data acquisition was carried out in mid atrial diastole. Table 1 specifies the imaging acquisition parameters. Some example images from this database can be seen in Fig. 1.

Table 1. Image acquisition

	CT	MRI
Scanner type	Philips Achieva 256 iCT	Philips 3T Achieva
Sequence	Angiography with ECG-gated and single breath hold	3D FLASH, respiratory gating and acquired at mid atrial diastole
TE, TR, TI	-	2.7 ms, 5.9 ms, 450–700 ms
Voxel in-plane	0.8 to 1 mm	1.4 mm
Slice thickness	0.4 mm	1.4 mm

Image acquisition parameters for the challenge CT and MRI data. Abbreviations: TE - Echo time, TR - Repetition time, TI - Inversion time.

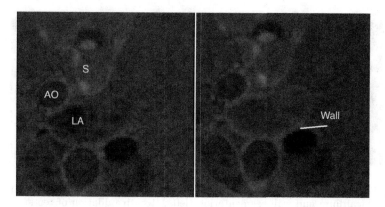

Fig. 1. MRI database: Example image from the image database (left) and its expert delineation of wall and blood pool chamber. Abbreviations: LA - left atrium, AO - Aorta, S - spine.

2.2 Atrial Wall Delineation

The atrial wall, in CT, was semi-automatically delineated by two observers with expertise on left atrial imaging. In the MRI datasets, these were manually delineated silce-by-slice by a single observer with good experience on atrial scans. The semi-automatic process on CT images consisted of a pixel-by-pixel dilation initiated from the atrial blood pool chamber. A single pixel dilation was compulsory followed by subsequent conditional dilations. These conditional dilations depended on a patient-specific atrial wall intensity range and thickness. This was followed by manual editing of the wall in each separate section of the image.

2.3 Evaluation of Wall Thickness

To study the performance of the algorithms submitted for the segmentation challenge, the binary segmentation masks obtained from each algorithm were analysed for left atrial wall thickness (LAWT). The thickness on the anterior and posterior sections of the LA were evaluated separately. In order to obtain LAWT from the binary masks an isotropic dilation process was implemented.

Determining LAWT from binary masks of the wall is not straightforward. Projecting and traversing normals from the inner boundary of the wall to its outer boundary to measure thickness has one important limitation. In regions of high curvature, the normals can be noisy resulting in misestimation of thickness. In [4], the authors highlighted these limitations and derived thickness from the length of field lines. These field lines were obtained from the Laplace solution that spanned the wall from the inner to the outer wall. In this work, a similar approach was undertaken by deriving such field lines using iterative isotropic dilation.

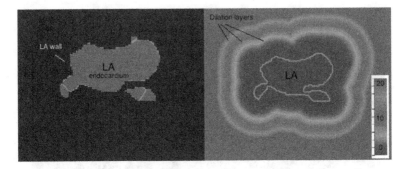

Fig. 2. This figure illustrates how the wall thickness is measured from binary masks of LA endocardium and wall segmentation (left). Iterative dilation of ten steps of the endocardial mask determines distance from each dilation layer (right).

Dilation was initiated from the endocardial mask and dilated by a single pixel in each direction, with up to ten iterative steps covering the entire possible width of the wall. Each *layer* of dilation of the endocardial mask determined the distance from the endocardium. Thus, the LAWT at all points on the LA wall masks could be measured by correspondence with the dilated layers of the endocardium. These steps are illustrated in Fig. 2.

2.4 Sectional Analysis of the Wall

The LAWT measured by each algorithm was evaluated on the posterior and anterior sections of the wall. The LA in each image was subdivided into these sections. The LAWT statistics in these sections were computed and compared between algorithms. Sectional analysis of the wall is relevant as several tissue based studies have highlighted regional differences in atrial wall thickness, even within superior and inferior aspects of the wall [5]. Different conclusions have been cited regarding comparative tissue thickness [6,7]. Figure 3 illustrates with an example how the wall was subdivided in this study.

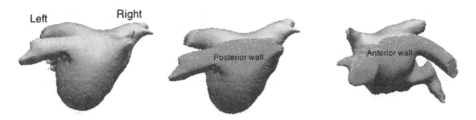

Fig. 3. The wall thickness was evaluated on the posterior and anterior sections of the wall. The image highlights these sections in the LA anatomy.

3   Results

Three research groups contributed to this challenge. These were INRIA Ascle-pios in France (INRA), Robarts Institute in Canada (ROBI) and Leiden University Medical Centre in The Netherlands (LUMC). INRA used region-growing to obtain the LA endocardium, followed by geodesic active contours for the LA epicardium. ROBI used intensity based thresholding by determining the threshold between ventricular myocardium and surrounding tissue. This was set at two standard deviations from the mean of myocardium intensity in Hounsfield units (HU). LUMC employed a multi-atlas registration of ten atlases for locating the LA chamber and pulmonary veins. A level-set evolution initiated from the LA chamber segmented the atrial wall based on the HU and incorporating prior knowledge of wall thickness.

The algorithms were evaluated and compared by computing the LAWT from their outputs. The expert delineations were also compared. The LAWT of the posterior wall computed on the CT images were (Mean $\pm$ SD): 1.1 ± 0.9 mm, 1.0 ± 0.7 mm, 1.6 ± 0.7 mm, 0.6 ± 0.2 mm for expert delineations, ROBI, INRA and LUMC respectively. For the anterior wall, the LAWT were (Mean $\pm$ SD): 0.9 ± 0.4 mm, 1.3 ± 0.9 mm, 1.7 ± 0.8 mm, 0.7 ± 0.3 mm for expert delineations, algorithms ROBI, INRA and LUMC respectively. Figure 4 provides a comparison in six separate cases. A sample segmentation from each algorithm is shown in Fig. 5.

The participating research groups did not choose to segment images from the MRI database. The expert delineations of the wall were evaluated by computing LAWT in five random images. The LAWT of the posterior wall computed on the MRI for the five separate images were (Mean $\pm$ SD): 2.1 ± 0.7 mm, 1.9 ± 0.7 mm, 1.8 ± 0.6 mm, 1.9 ± 0.8 mm, 1.9 ± 0.7 mm. The LAWT of the anterior wall computed in the five separate images were (Mean $\pm$ SD): 1.9 ± 0.7 mm, 1.5 ± 0.6 mm, 1.7 ± 0.7 mm, 1.6 ± 0.7 mm, 1.8 ± 0.9 mm. The comparison of LAWT in the five cases is shown in Fig. 6.

4   Discussions

There is good agreement between the algorithms and expert delineations on the posterior wall. The exception is LUMC which under-estimates the thickness in most cases. However, there is good agreement between LUMC and the expert delineation on the anterior wall. Both ROBI and INRA report greater thickness for the anterior wall. The posterior wall is found to be generally thicker than the anterior wall in the CT scans. This has also been reported in some meta studies [8]. Some algorithms have imposed a minimum thickness constraint, usually one pixel (i.e. 0.4 mm), resulting in the slightly skewed box-plots.

The range of LAWT values measured with MRI was in close agreement with CT, both for the posterior and anterior walls. The MRI and CT images were not from the same patients. For a more extensive analysis of LAWT in MRI, refer to [9].

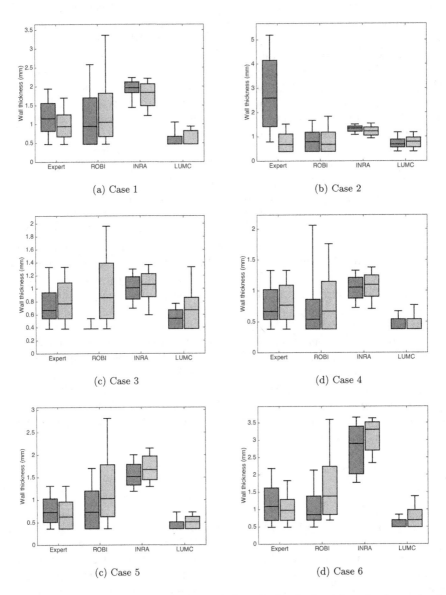

Fig. 4. Sectional wall thickness analysis of the submitted algorithms in six randomly selected CT images from the database. In each sub-plot, the bars to the left and right represent posterior and anterior walls respectively.

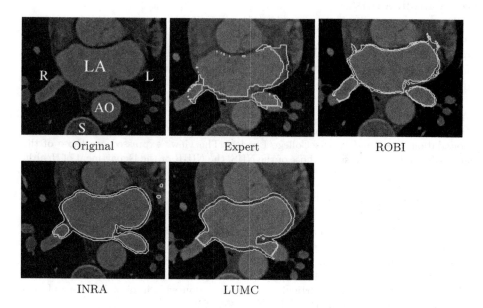

Original   Expert   ROBI

INRA   LUMC

Fig. 5. One example from the CT database comparing segmentations of the atrial wall in the expert delineation and the submitted algorithms. Abbreviations: L - left side, R - right side, LA - left atrium, AO - Aorta, S - spine.

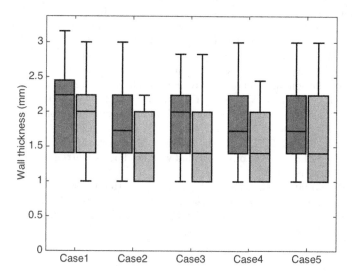

Fig. 6. Wall thickness in expert delineations of five randomly selected MRI images from the challenge image database

5 Conclusions

This work collates results of the algorithms on the image database released for quantification of atrial wall thickness. To our knowledge, this database is the first of its kind for left atrial wall. Future work will provide an extensive analysis of the algorithm results.

Acknowledgements. This research was supported by the National Institute for Health Research (NIHR) Biomedical Research Centre at Guy's and St Thomas' NHS Foundation Trust and King's College London. The views expressed are those of the author(s) and not necessarily those of the NHS, the NIHR or the Department of Health.

References

1. Feinberg, W.M., Blackshear, J.L., Laupacis, A., Kronmal, R., Hart, R.G.: Prevalence, age distribution, and gender of patients with atrial fibrillation: analysis and implications. Arch. Intern. Med. **155**(5), 469–473 (1995)
2. Cabrera, J.A., Ho, S.Y., Climent, V., Sánchez-Quintana, D.: The architecture of the left lateral atrial wall: a particular anatomic region with implications for ablation of atrial fibrillation. Eur. Heart J. **29**(3), 356–362 (2008)
3. López-Candales, A., Grewal, H., Katz, W.: The importance of increased interatrial septal thickness in patients with atrial fibrillation: a transesophageal echocardiographic study. Echocardiography **22**(5), 408–414 (2005)
4. Bishop, M., Rajani, R., Plank, G., Gaddum, N., Carr-White, G., Wright, M., O'Neill, M., Niederer, S.: Three-dimensional atrial wall thickness maps to inform catheter ablation procedures for atrial fibrillation. Europace **18**(3), 376–383 (2016)
5. Sánchez-Quintana, D., Cabrera, J.A., Climent, V., Farré, J., de Mendonça, M.C., Ho, S.Y.: Anatomic relations between the esophagus and left atrium and relevance for ablation of atrial fibrillation. Circulation **112**(10), 1400–1405 (2005)
6. Hall, B., Jeevanantham, V., Simon, R., Filippone, J., Vorobiof, G., Daubert, J.: Variation in left atrial transmural wall thickness at sites commonly targeted for ablation of atrial fibrillation. J. Intervent. Card. Electrophysiol. **17**(2), 127–132 (2006)
7. Platonov, P.G., Ivanov, V., Ho, S.Y., Mitrofanova, L.: Left atrial posterior wall thickness in patients with and without atrial fibrillation: data from 298 consecutive autopsies. J. Cardiovasc. Electrophysiol. **19**(7), 689–692 (2008)
8. Whitaker, J., Rajani, R., Chubb, H., Gabrawi, M., Varela, M., Wright, M., Niederer, S., O'Neill, M.D.: The role of myocardial wall thickness in atrial arrhythmogenesis. Europace, euw014 (2016)
9. Varela, M., Kolbitsch, C., Theron, A., Morgan, R., Henningsson, M., Schaeffter, T., Aslanidi, O.: 3D high-resolution atrial wall thickness maps using black-blood psir. J. Cardiovasc. Magn. Reson. (Suppl.) **17** (2015). Society of Magnetic Resonance Imaging (SCMR)

Left Atrial Wall Segmentation Using Clinically Correlated Metrics

Jiro Inoue[(⊠)] and Maria Drangova

Robarts Research Institute, Western University, London, Canada
jinoue@robarts.ca

Abstract. The thickness of the left atrium wall may be an important parameter in atrial fibrillation disease mechanisms and subsequent treatment by catheter ablation. We have previously developed a simple, threshold-based, direct wall thickness measure from CT that has been found to correlate with clinical outcomes. In this paper, we describe the application of this method to the segmentation of the left atrium wall in the 2016 STACOM Left Atrium Wall Thickness Challenge.

Our original method sought to partially automate the way a clinical researcher manually measures left atrial wall thickness to increase precision and repeatability. We have adapted our method to create a segmented volume instead of individual measurements in order to meet the challenge goals. We apply the method to the ten contrast-enhanced CT images provided.

Keywords: Left atrium · Wall thickness · Segmentation · CT

1 Introduction

Left atrial (LA) wall thickness (LAWT) may be an important parameter in the treatment of atrial fibrillation by catheter ablation [1, 2]. The aim of catheter ablation is to create transmural lesions in the LA wall, which then heal into non-conductive scar tissue. One suspected mechanism for ablation failure is lack of transmurality in the formed lesions due to thicker-than-expected atrial wall tissue. LAWT has also been implicated in the mechanism of atrial fibrillation [3].

LAWT can be measured directly [1, 2] or by first segmenting, and measuring the segmented volume [4–6]. However, no method of LAWT measurement has been strongly validated. There is a need to standardize and validate LAWT measurement methods in order to translate this parameter into clinical use.

The 2016 STACOM left atrial wall thickness challenge is a collaborative challenge with the primary objective of exploring the segmentation of a standard set of cardiac CT and MR images, and the secondary objective of measuring LAWT. In this study, we only consider the CT image data.

Segmentation of the LA wall is challenging for multiple reasons. The thickness of the atrial is roughly 1–3 mm [7–9], which is similar to the resolution of clinical MR images – the challenge data has an isotropic 1.4 mm resolution. Clinical CT images have slightly better voxel spacing – approximately 0.5 mm in the axial plane. Image quality is often poor, with low signal-to-noise ratios, and various imaging artifacts from

© Springer International Publishing AG 2017
T. Mansi et al. (Eds.): STACOM 2016, LNCS 10124, pp. 201–210, 2017.
DOI: 10.1007/978-3-319-52718-5_22

sources such as gating errors and implanted metallic devices. Cardiac anatomy is also challenging since cardiac morphology varies from patient-to-patient, and extra-cardiac structures can be difficult to distinguish from the heart itself.

We have previously developed a simple, threshold-based, direct wall thickness measure from CT that was found to correlate with clinical outcomes [10]. A limitation of this method is that the point-based methodology is not designed to generate a segmentation of the entire atrial wall – locations with inconclusive results were manually excluded. In this work, we adapt this method to the challenge format by modifying it to incorporate more automation, and to generate a segmentation based on the point-based thickness measurements. Atrial thickness maps and segmentation are generated for the ten CT data sets provided.

2   Methods

2.1   CT Images and Pre-processing

The challenge data consisted of ten contrast-enhanced CT images. Segmented LA blood pool and eroded LA blood pool volumes were also provided.

For each data set, a patient-specific tissue intensity model was created by sampling regions of left atrial blood pool and ventricular myocardium, as shown in Fig. 1. For both tissue types, the image intensity means and standard deviations were collected and from these samples, two thresholds are calculated: the threshold between blood and myocardium is calculated as the mean of the image intensities of these two tissues, and the threshold between myocardium and surrounding tissue is calculated as two standard deviations below the mean myocardium intensity. The eroded blood pool volume was also meshed to create a base 3D geometry of the blood pool. Pre-processing was performed using ITK-SNAP [11].

2.2   LAWT Measure

Our LAWT measure seeks to emulate the way a clinical researcher manually measures LAWT, augmented with computerized precision and repeatability. The fundamental principle is to distinguish the atrial wall based on image intensity (thresholding) with manual vetting of misclassification, and averaging multiple measurements with outlier removal. For the purposes of this study, manual vetting was not performed, and the method was adapted for image segmentation by converting thickness measurements into a labeled volume. A graph neighbourhood-based smoothing operator was used instead of outlier removal and anatomical region-based averaging.

LAWT is first calculated on a point-by-point basis on a mesh of the LA blood pool. Using the provided eroded blood pool segmentation, a 3D mesh was constructed and a line was projected from each mesh vertex, in the direction of the vertex normal. A line segment extending from 5 mm inside the mesh to 10 mm was defined and the CT

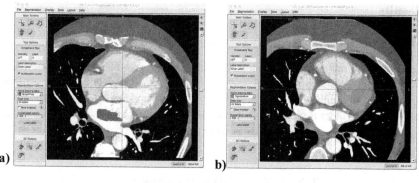

Fig. 1. Sampling the image intensities in in the left atrium blood pool and myocardium. (a) Left atrial blood pool sample. (b) Myocardium sample taken from left ventricle. (c) Image statistics on samples: mean and standard deviations used for patient-specific tissue intensity model.

image was resampled along this line at 0.1 mm intervals using trilinear interpolation to create an intensity profile along this line. The distance from the eroded mesh to the first blood pool/myocardium (endocardial) crossing to the first myocardium/surroundings (epicardial) crossings was recorded for each vertex.

The original method included averaging and outlier removal based on multiple measurements – this step was approximated by automated smoothing. A 2-neighbourhood vertex-based averaging operation was defined to smooth the measurements. This was applied twice for the endocardial crossings and five times for the epicardial crossings.

For each vertex in the eroded mesh, the thickness was calculated as the distance between the two crossings after smoothing. For visualization purposes, thicknesses were mapped to the surface of the eroded blood pool mesh for each patient. These smoothed crossing points were also used to dilate the eroded mesh to create separate endocardial and epicardial meshes. The segmented atrial wall was defined as the region that lay between the two meshes. Thickness measurement and segmentation were implemented using C++ and MeVisLab (MeVis Medical Solutions AG, Germany).

3   Results

3.1   Image Characteristics

Baseline image characteristics of the ten CT images are shown in Table 1. There was a wide variation in both contrast level and noise in the images. Additionally, artifacts were present in a number of images. Images 5 and 6 appeared to be identical CT volumes although the provided eroded blood pool segmentations differed. For the purposes of this study, these two images were processed independently.

Table 1. Baseline image characteristics.

Patient	Axial res. (mm)	Slice thick. (mm)	Blood mean (HU)	Blood S.D (HU)	Myo. mean (HU)	Myo. S.D. (HU)	Artifacts
1	0.47	0.39	293.6	37.0	73.1	16.2	a
2	0.43	0.45	653.3	51.3	124.4	37.5	b
3	0.39	0.45	589.6	35.6	178.1	36.7	a
4	0.46	0.40	344.4	40.0	77.9	23.2	a
5*	0.38	0.45	241.1	42.6	115.7	31.1	b, c, d
6*	0.38	0.45	252.9	53.9	117.3	34.5	b, c
7	0.36	0.45	624.3	55.9	90.5	48.2	
8	0.49	0.45	486.6	31.2	86.5	25.9	
9	0.49	0.45	530.0	29.8	95.7	21.8	
10	0.41	0.40	406.7	93.5	111.3	45.6	b, d

Types of artifaces: [a]Gating artifact. [b]Wires/leads/device. [c]Uneven contrast in LA. [d]Eroded segmentation missing top of atrium. *Volumes 5 and 6 are identical cases, but differed in the provided eroded blood pool segmentations.

3.2   LAWT Measures

Thickness-mapped LA meshes are shown in Fig. 2. The accuracy of these measurements cannot be established but certain trends are apparent. In the majority of cases, there is excessive thickening near the center of the posterior wall, corresponding to the expected location of the esophagus. There also appear to be errors near the ends of the pulmonary veins, especially the right superior, where the pulmonary artery crosses over the LA. These locations are less concerning, as they are not typically ablated.

The anterior wall of the LA has more complex geometry, as it is lies internal to the heart and lies adjacent to the right atrium aorta and intracardiac structures. Two examples are shown in Fig. 3. The region adjacent to the right atrium (bottom left

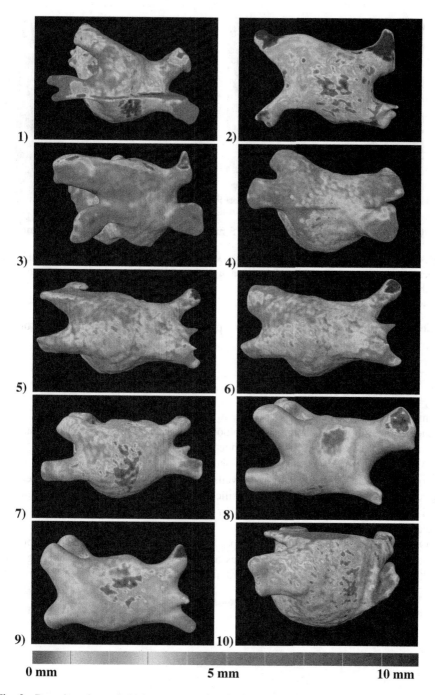

Fig. 2. Posterior view of thickness-mapped atrial left atria. Images labeled as per original challenge data numbers. Dark red regions are excessively thick and likely the result of measurement errors. The central posterior wall is often adjacent to the esophagus, and difficult to segment. (Color figure online)

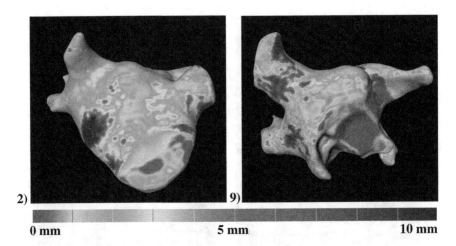

Fig. 3. Anterior view of two thickness-mapped left atria. Images labeled as per original challenge data numbers. The bottom left region in the image lies adjacent to the right atrium, and usually exhibits uneven contrast.

section of each image) is particularly error prone due to differences in contrast, but is generally not a candidate for ablation.

3.3   Segmentation Results

Examples of the segmentations are shown in Fig. 4. In most cases, the atrial wall segmentations follow the contour of the blood pool, as expected. Overall segmentation accuracy was not evaluated at this time due to lack of a gold standard.

Areas corresponding to thickening as seen on the thickness-mapped meshes show obvious errors on the segmentation as well. In many of the segmented volumes, an excessive number of islands of misclassification were present inside the regions of atrial wall label. This is likely due to either degeneracies in the endocardial and epicardial meshes, or numerical errors.

Of particular interest is the blood pool contrast in patient 5/6, which appears unusually uneven. Since the tissue classes are largely separated by thresholding, this resulted in jagged endocardial and epicardial boundaries; effect shown in Fig. 5.

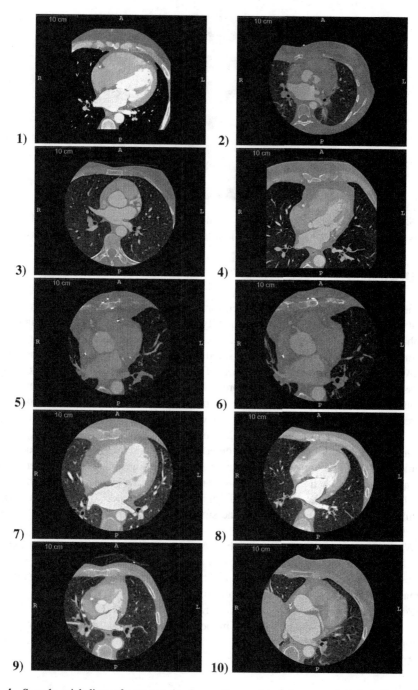

Fig. 4. Sample axial slices of segmented volumes. Images labeled as per original challenge data numbers. Pixels identified as atrial wall are shown in red. Specific areas of obvious errors (very thick walls) often include regions adjacent to the right atrium, near the mitral valve and esophagus. (Color figure online)

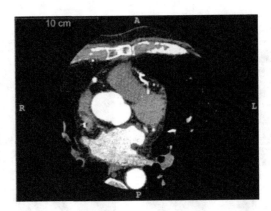

Fig. 5. CT image number 6 with narrow windowing (window: 443 HU, level: −114 HU). Uneven contrast in the left atrium resulted in jagged endocardial (and epicardial) boundaries.

4 Discussion

Segmentations were successfully derived for all ten CT data sets, but the segmentation quality was highly variable. Image quality, anatomical difficulties (especially the esophagus, and the conversion from thickness measurement all introduced errors into the final segmentation results. While standard post-processing steps such as island removal may allow the correction of some of these errors, large-scale problems such as excessively jagged boundaries are more difficult resolve. Image intensity levels for various tissues vary considerably. This is particularly apparently in the blood pool, where the level of circulating contrast can vary, resulting in patient-to-patient differences of up to several hundred Hounsfield units.

Due to the sampling method of determining boundaries between tissues, our technique is sensitive to non-uniform contrast in the left atrium. While this sensitivity may be acceptable when making expert-supervised individual measurements, the errors may be problematic for an automated segmentation method. The esophagus, right atrium and other intra- and extra-cardiac structures can also introduce errors into the segmentation.

While it is clear that some areas of the LA are more difficult to segment than others, the relevance of these areas is less clear. Not all regions of the LA are regularly ablated. Thus, averages and Dice metrics may not be meaningful measures of LA wall segmentation, if applied to the entire left atrium.

Potential applications of a robust, accurate LAWT measurement include the creation of a prescriptive ablation-dosing model that takes patient anatomy into consideration. Accurate methodology may also facilitate scientific investigation of LAWT as it correlates with cardiac disease processes.

4.1 Limitations

Smoothing parameters were arbitrarily selected and applied uniformly to all data sets. Thus, results are not indicative of optimality using this framework. The conversion from thickness map to segmentation is also error prone due to possible degeneracies in the underlying 3D meshes. Many of the small errors in the segmented atrial wall volumes may be due to the conversion process rather than the LAWT measurement method.

5 Conclusion

Qualitatively, our method generated plausible segmentation and thickness measurement (<5 mm) results in most cases, but quantitatively validating the accuracy of the method was not possible due to the lack of an objective ground truth. The compiled STACOM challenge results may provide insight into the validation accuracy.

Some obvious errors such as small islands in the segmented volume are correctable through standard post-processing techniques such as island removal or regularization. Other errors such highly jagged boundaries or misclassification of the esophagus may be more difficult to correct. More robust handling of noisy images and variations in internal contrast may improve the performance in low quality images and independent segmentation and removal of the esophagus before atrial wall segmentation may also improve results in many cases.

Acknowledgements. This research was funded in part by Canadian Institutes for Health Research (CIHR) grant #27790.

References

1. Suenari, K., Nakano, Y., Hirai, Y., Ogi, H., Oda, N., Makita, Y., Ueda, S., Kajihara, K., Tokuyama, T., Motoda, C., Fujiwara, M., Chayama, K., Kihara, Y.: Left atrial thickness under the catheter ablation lines in patients with paroxysmal atrial fibrillation: insights from 64-slice multidetector computed tomography. Heart Vessels **28**, 360–368 (2012)
2. Takahashi, K., Okumura, Y., Watanabe, I., Nagashima, K., Sonoda, K., Sasaki, N., Kogawa, R., Iso, K., Ohkubo, K., Nakai, T., Hirayama, A.: Relation between left atrial wall thickness in patients with atrial fibrillation and intracardiac electrogram characteristics and atp-provoked dormant pulmonary vein conduction. J. Cardiovasc. Electrophysiol. **26**, 597–605 (2015)
3. Wi, J., Lee, H.J., Uhm, J.S., Kim, J.Y., Pak, H.N., Lee, M., Kim, Y.J., Joung, B.: Complex fractionated atrial electrograms related to left atrial wall thickness. J. Cardiovasc. Electrophysiol. **25**, 1141–1149 (2014)
4. Koppert, M., Rongen, P.M., Prokop, M., ter Haar Romeny, B.M., van Assen, H.C.: Cardiac left atrium CT image segmentation for ablation guidance. In: 2010 IEEE International Symposium on Biomedical Imaging: From Nano to Macro, pp. 480–483. IEEE (2010)
5. Inoue, J., Skanes, A.C., White, J.A., Rajchl, M., Drangova, M.: Patient-specific left atrial wall-thickness measurement and visualization for radiofrequency ablation. In: SPIE Medical Imaging, 90361N-90361N-90366 (2014)

6. Inoue, J., Baxter, John, S.,H., Drangova, M.: Left atrial wall segmentation from CT for radiofrequency catheter ablation planning. In: Oyarzun Laura, C., Shekhar, R., Wesarg, S., González Ballester, M.Á., Drechsler, K., Sato, Y., Erdt, M., Linguraru, M.G. (eds.) CLIP 2015. LNCS, vol. 9401, pp. 71–78. Springer, Heidelberg (2016). doi:10.1007/978-3-319-31808-0_9

7. Hall, B., Jeevanantham, V., Simon, R., Filippone, J., Vorobiof, G., Daubert, J.: Variation in left atrial transmural wall thickness at sites commonly targeted for ablation of atrial fibrillation. J. Interv. Card. Electrophysiol. 17, 127–132 (2006)

8. Ho, S.Y., Sanchez-Quintana, D., Cabrera, J.A., Anderson, R.H.: Anatomy of the left atrium: implications for radiofrequency ablation of atrial fibrillation. J. Cardiovasc. Electrophysiol. 10, 1525–1533 (1999)

9. Sanchez-Quintana, D., Cabrera, J.A., Climent, V., Farre, J., Mendonca, M.C., Ho, S.Y.: Anatomic relations between the esophagus and left atrium and relevance for ablation of atrial fibrillation. Circulation 112, 1400–1405 (2005)

10. Inoue, J., Skanes, A.C., Gula, L.J., Drangova, M.: Effect of left atrial wall thickness on radiofrequency ablation success. J. Cardiovasc. Electrophysiol. 27, 1298–1303 (2016)

11. Yushkevich, P.A., Piven, J., Hazlett, H.C., Smith, R.G., Ho, S., Gee, J.C., Gerig, G.: User-guided 3D active contour segmentation of anatomical structures: significantly improved efficiency and reliability. Neuroimage 31, 1116–1128 (2006)

STACOM-SLAWT Challenge: Left Atrial Wall Segmentation and Thickness Measurement Using Region Growing and Marker-Controlled Geodesic Active Contour

Shuman Jia[1]($\boxtimes$), Loïc Cadour[1], Hubert Cochet[2], and Maxime Sermesant[1]

[1] University of Côte d'Azur, Asclepios Research Group, Inria, Sophia Antipolis, France
shuman.jia@inria.fr
[2] IHU Liryc, University of Bordeaux, Pessac, France

Abstract. Analyzing the structure of the left atrium can provide precious insights into the pathology of atrial fibrillation, eventually resulting in optimization of treatment plans. In this paper, an interactive and patient-specific method is presented to segment the left atrial endocardium(We refer to the segmentation of the region inside the left atrial endocardium as the segmentation of the left atrial endocardium, the same for epicardium.), the left atrial epicardium and measure the left atrial wall thickness from cardiac computed tomography images. A region growing algorithm was adapted to segment the left atrial endocardium, whereas the left atrial epicardium was segmented indirectly: a marker-controlled geodesic active contour model was defined on its surrounding environment. The results of the left atrial wall thickness were then mapped onto meshes generated from the endocardium segmentation. We tested our pipeline on 10 datasets as a part of the STACOM 2016 Left Atrial Wall Segmentation Challenge and we compared our method with manual segmentation. Aimed at facilitating the segmentation of the left atrial thin-wall structure, this pipeline is partially implemented in MUSIC software for clinical use. The expertise of clinicians can be added through the choice of specific parameters for each patient, although this remains optional owing to the robustness of the approach.

Keywords: Atrial fibrillation · Left atrial wall thickness · 3-Dimensional image segmentation · Cardiac computed tomography (CT) · Region growing · Geodesic active contour

1 Introduction

Atrial fibrillation (AF) is the most common type of cardiac arrhythmia, characterized by uncoordinated electrical activation and disorganized contraction of the atria. Around 2% to 3% of the population in Europe and North America, as of

© Springer International Publishing AG 2017
T. Mansi et al. (Eds.): STACOM 2016, LNCS 10124, pp. 211–219, 2017.
DOI: 10.1007/978-3-319-52718-5_23

2014, were affected, and its prevalence rate is increasing worldwide [1]. This epidemic, with or without symptoms, is likely to be associated with life-threatening consequences, including heart failure, heart attack and stroke.

Atrial ablation, an effective treatment for AF, may be recommended for drug refractory patients. This invasive procedure establishes transmural lesions to block the arrhythmia while avoiding impairing extra-cardiac tissues. Thereby the radio-frequency power dose, delivered for ablation during the procedure, relies on local myocardial thickness, which demonstrates variations by region and by subject [2,3]. Reduction of left atrial (LA) wall thickness also appears in AF patients when compared with controls, according to study by autopsy [4].

Model-based segmentation and region growing approach have been tested on the segmentation of the left atrium [5,6]. Furthermore, several methods have been developed to measure automatically the LA wall thickness from computed tomography (CT) images. In [7], a segmentation of the wall on four regions, inter-atrial septum, below right inferior pulmonary vein, appendage and anterior wall, was performed whereas [8,9] chose to build a pipeline based on multi-region segmentation method. However, this task remains challenging, because the LA wall is heterogeneous, possibly consisting of fat granules and fibrosis, especially in patients of myocardial diseases or persistent AF. The accuracy of the segmentation is also difficult to validate, as few manual segmentations or reliable ground truths are available.

In this paper, we present an interactive pipeline to segment the LA wall and measure the wall thickness from cardiac CT images. The expertise of clinicians can be introduced through the choice of parameters. Compared to previous works, we propose an inverse way to segment the LA thin-wall structure. The segmentation was divided into 2 parts, LA endocardium and LA epicardium. The former was segmented with high accuracy using region growing combined with patient-specific intensity value threshold. The latter was segmented indirectly from its surrounding environment, to address the fuzzy boundaries problem. Algorithms employed were in 3-dimensional (3D) space.

The rest of the paper is organized as follows: we summarize our method using a flowchart in Sect. 2, along with detailed illustration of region growing and marker-controlled geodesic active contour algorithms. Results and evaluation are shown in Sect. 3, and a discussion of the limitations of this study in Sect. 4.

2   Materials and Methods

2.1   Data Acquisition and Pre-processing

The method was applied to a database consisting of 10 3D CT image datasets, provided by the STACOM Left Atrial Wall Thickness Challenge.

Coronary Computed Tomography Angiography (CCTA) was performed on a Philips 256 iCT scanner. All patients were injected with an intravenous contrast agent. The scans were ECG-gated in a single breath hold. The images were acquired at 0.5 mm in-plane resolution with a slice thickness of 1 mm, and reconstructed to a 0.8 to 1.0 mm slice thickness with a 0.4 mm slice increment and a 250 mm field of view. The image matrix was kept at 512×512 matrix, constructed with a sharp reconstruction kernel [10]. The pixel values were in Hounsfield units (HU).

The images were manually cropped around the region of interest, namely the left atrium. The intensity values outside the range from $-500\ HU$ to $500\ HU$ were set to nearer bound, so as to obtain a better visualization of blood pool, muscles and fat within the region that was meant to be segmented.

2.2 Methodology

We summarize our method into following steps, as shows the flowchart in Fig. 1:

1. Drawing polygons on axial slices of CT images to isolate the left atrium[1].
2. Sampling intensity values of blood and muscles.
3. Segmenting the LA endocardium using region growing according to intensity values statistics.
4. Thresholding neighboring tissues (fat, other blood pools) of the LA wall.
5. Segmenting the LA epicardium using geodesic active contour based on markers of neighboring tissues.
6. Calculating distance map of the LA epicardium segmentation.
7. Mapping the distance onto meshes of the LA endocardium.

Currently most steps are implemented in MUSIC software (multimodality software for specific imaging in cardiology, developed by *IHU Liryc, University of Bordeaux* and *Inria Sophia Antipolis*) [11].

2.3 Region Growing

We chose one pixel inside the left atrium, a connected component, as seed. The seed was raised into a gowning region. Neighboring pixels next to the growing region whose intensity values fell within a certain range were considered part of the left atrium. The region evolved iteratively until no more pixel was assigned.

To determine whether a pixel belonged to the left atrium, statistical analysis was performed on intensity values of tissues samples. Given the histogram of muscles samples and blood samples, we computed the mean and standard deviation of intensity values, for muscles $I(\mu, \sigma^2)$ and for blood $I'(\mu', \sigma'^2)$. Then we set a threshold to distinguish these two classes as

$$th = \frac{\mu\sigma' + \mu'\sigma}{\sigma + \sigma'}. \tag{1}$$

Neighbor pixels of the growing region with intensity values upper than the threshold th were assigned to the left atrium. Accordingly, spatial constraint and user-provided intensity information are combined in the algorithm.

---

[1] For step 1, polygons were drawn manually on a dozen of slices for each case and then interpolated automatically on the rest. Images are shown in axial planes.

To further negate the impact of noise in original CT images, alternating sequential filters (ASFs) were used to post-process the LA endocardium segmentation. This step is compulsory for CT images with low quality. Alternating sequential filters are composed of pairs of idempotent morphological filters with structuring elements of increasing sizes. They extract the geometrical characteristics and minimize the distortion of objects [12,13]. In our experiment, we used pairs of closing and opening with structuring elements of increasing radius from 0.25 mm, 0.50 mm to 0.75 mm sequentially.

2.4   Marker-Controlled Geodesic Active Contour (MCGAC)

Geodesic active contour algorithm [14], represents contour as zero crossing of a level-set function. An initial contour propagates to touch the shape boundaries, as the level-set function progresses in time until

$$\frac{\partial u}{\partial t} = 0, \tag{2}$$

where u is the level-set function under following conditions:

$$u|_{t=0} = u_0 \tag{3a}$$

$$\frac{\partial u}{\partial t} = g(c + \kappa)|\nabla u| + \nabla u \nabla g, \tag{3b}$$

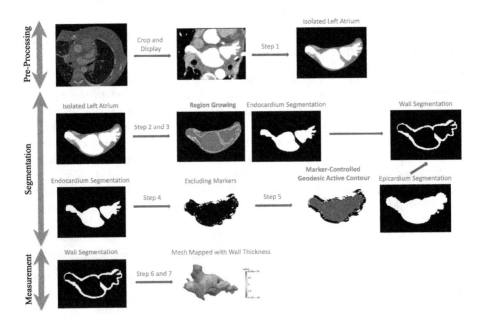

Fig. 1. The flowchart of our method.

where u_0 is the initial level-set function; c is a constant to provide a steady velocity; κ is related to the curvature of the level-set function as $\kappa = div(\frac{\nabla u}{|\nabla u|})$; g is an edge detector function of image, which is strictly decreasing towards the outside of the region to be segmented and has values near 0 at the boundary to stop the evolution of curves.

In Eq. 3b, three terms affect the way that a level-set function evolves:

- Advection term: $gc|\nabla u|$, related to progression speed of curves.
- Curvature term: $g\kappa|\nabla u|$, related to curvature of curves.
- Propagation term: $\nabla u \nabla g$, related to expansion of curves.

The algorithm is implemented in Insight Segmentation and Registration Toolkit (ITK), which uses three parameters (advection, curvature and propagation scaling, noted here as S_a, S_c and S_p) to assign weighting ratios to each term and adjust their influence in the evolution process of the level-set function. We chose manually $S_a = 10 \times S_c = S_p = 5$. The initial level-set function u_0 was computed as a distance map of the LA endocardium segmentation. The edge detector function g was simply set to 0 on excluded regions and 1 on the rest of the image.

As for excluded regions, neighboring tissues other than muscles outside the LA wall were marked as excluded for the segmentation. Since CT images display relative linear attenuation values of tissues, and correspond to Hounsfield units (HU) scale, they may be used to characterize tissues [15]. Based on approximate HU values for air (-1000), fat (-100 to -50), muscle (10 to 50) and blood (300 to 400), we set 0 HU as upper threshold for fat (and air) and th, as defined in Eq. 1, as lower threshold for blood. Besides, fat granules of size smaller than $1\,mm^3$ were regarded as inside the LA wall, thus not excluded. Margins were kept to avoid misleading markers resulting from noise or density variation. Lastly, all pixels further than 6 mm away from the left atrium were also excluded, according to studies of the LA wall thickness on excised hearts [2,3].

The markers of neighboring tissues were introduced to address the fuzzy boundaries problem, as the intensity gradient between the LA wall and its neighboring tissues is small and noise may blur original CT images. Then we adapted geodesic active contour model based on excluding markers, because the LA wall may be attached to muscles belonging to other organs such as esophagus, aorta, lung etc., and hence cannot be segmented only based on intensity information. Geodesic active contour, on the other hand, involves curvature constraint of shape to solve this problem.

3   Results

3.1   Parameters

Parameter setting mentioned in Sect. 2 can be altered depending on cases, but in this study we followed the same rule for all 10 cases to test the robustness of the algorithm with respect to different inputs.

Intensity value thresholds th used during region growing process are shown in Table 1.

Table 1. Intensity value thresholds used for 10 datasets tested.

Dataset	#1	#2	#3	#4	#5
Threshold th	224.3 HU	419.5 HU	485.7 HU	226.6 HU	131.6 HU
Dataset	#6	#7	#8	#9	#10
Threshold th	136 HU	448.2 HU	358.4 HU	345.8 HU	267.1 HU

3.2   Left Atrial Wall Segmentation

Here we present preliminary results of the LA wall segmentation, and comparison with manual segmentation, as shown in Fig. 2.

The proposed method closely approximated the wall thickness, as compared with manual segmentation. Differences lay in the segmentation of the anterior LA wall, which is not fully involved in the manual segmentation provided. The intersecting surfaces inside pulmonary veins and on mitral valve are presented in our segmentation with rather thinner wall, which should not have been included.

Remark. We segmented the LA appendage and pulmonary veins connected to the left atrium as well, which is different from the manual segmentation provided.

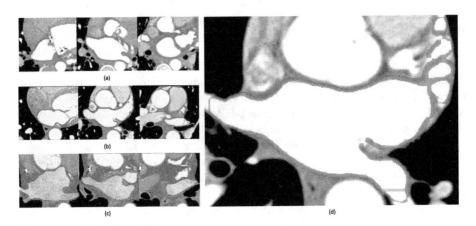

Fig. 2. Axial slices of CT images, overlapped with manual segmentation of the left atrial wall in green, our segmentation in red, intersection of the two in chartreuse. (a) Dataset #2; (b) dataset #3; (c) dataset #5; (d) example slice zoomed in. (Color figure online)

3.3   Wall Thickness Measurement

We computed the LA wall thickness using the nearest distance from each point on the LA endocardium to the LA epicardium. Meshes of the LA endocardium were generated using The Visualization Toolkit (VTK).

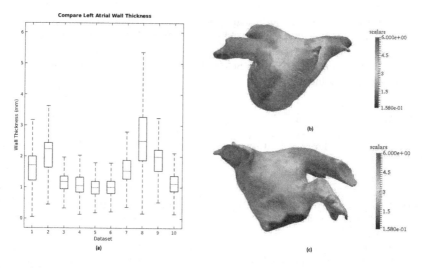

Fig. 3. (a) Mean and interquartile range of the left atrial wall thickness for 10 datasets tested, with maximum whisker length specified as 1.5 times the interquartile range; (b) left atrial wall thickness map for dataset #8, posterior view; (c) left atrial wall thickness map for dataset #8, anterior view.

The LA wall thickness varies by subject as well as by region, as shown in Fig. 3. From the mean and range of the wall thickness, we can see that dataset #8 has a thicker LA wall compared with other datasets, whereas dataset #5 and #6 have a thinner LA wall. The results for dataset #8 are shown as an example.

Alternating sequential filters may be used to post-process the segmentation results. The LA epicardium segmentation, using marker-controlled geodesic active contour, takes into account the heterogeneity of the LA wall, and therefore can have small granules excluded. Whether or not to smooth the contour of the LA epicardium, depends on how the LA wall is defined.

4 Conclusion

We proposed a new method to segment the LA wall, making use of patient-specific intensity value information and surrounding environment of the LA wall. Despite good match of wall thickness with manual segmentation, the accuracy of the segmentation is still hard to validate as few reliable ground truths are available.

Although the study reached its aims, there exist some limitations to be mentioned. The proposed MCGAC method, applying uniform parameters to all subregions of the LA wall, cannot achieve a region-wise constraint on curvature, which could lead to incorrectly assigned pixels. Potential future work to improve the accuracy of this work: further eliminating the influence of noise; region-wise segmentation based on different surrounding environment of LA sub-regions; parameters testing; combining measurement approaches [16] and minimizing measurement error of the wall thickness.

Acknowledgments. Part of the research was funded by the *Agence Nationale de la Recherche (ANR)*/ERA CoSysMed SysAFib and ANR MIGAT projects. The authors would like to thank Marc-Michel Rohé and Hervé Delingette for their constructive feedback and *Inria dtk team* (Nicolas Schnitzler and Thibaud Kloczko) for helping in implementing the pipeline.

References

1. Zoni-Berisso, M., Lercari, F., Carazza, T., Domenicucci, S., et al.: Epidemiology of atrial fibrillation: European perspective. Clin. Epidemiol **6**, 213–220 (2014). doi:10.2147/CLEP.S47385

2. Ho, S.Y., Sanchez-Quintana, D., Cabrera, J.A., Anderson, R.H.: Anatomy of the left atrium: implications for radiofrequency ablation of atrial fibrillation. J. Cardiovasc. Electrophysiol. **10**(11), 1525–1533 (1999). doi:10.1111/j.1540-8167.1999.tb00211.x

3. Sánchez-Quintana, D., Cabrera, J.A., Climent, V., Farré, J., de Mendonça, M.C., Ho, S.Y.: Anatomic relations between the esophagus and left atrium and relevance for ablation of atrial fibrillation. Circulation **112**(10), 1400–1405 (2005). doi:10.1161/CIRCULATIONAHA.105.551291

4. Hassink, R.J., Aretz, H.T., Ruskin, J., Keane, D.: Morphology of atrial myocardium in human pulmonary veins: a postmortem analysis in patients with and without atrial fibrillation. J. Am. Coll. Cardiol. **42**(6), 1108–1114 (2003). doi:10.1016/S0735-1097(03)00918-5

5. Tobon-Gomez, C., Peters, J., Weese, J., Pinto, K., Karim, R., Schaeffter, T., Razavi, R., Rhode, K.S.: Left atrial segmentation challenge: a unified benchmarking framework. In: Camara, O., Mansi, T., Pop, M., Rhode, K., Sermesant, M., Young, A. (eds.) STACOM 2013. LNCS, vol. 8330, pp. 1–13. Springer, Heidelberg (2014). doi:10.1007/978-3-642-54268-8_1

6. Kutra, D., Saalbach, A., Lehmann, H., Groth, A., Dries, S.P.M., Krueger, M.W., Dössel, O., Weese, J.: Automatic multi-model-based segmentation of the left atrium in cardiac MRI scans. In: Ayache, N., Delingette, H., Golland, P., Mori, K. (eds.) MICCAI 2012. LNCS, vol. 7511, pp. 1–8. Springer, Heidelberg (2012). doi:10.1007/978-3-642-33418-4_1

7. Dewland, T.A., Wintermark, M., Vaysman, A., Smith, L.M., Tong, E., Vittinghoff, E., Marcus, G.M.: Use of computed tomography to identify atrial fibrillation associated differences in left atrial wall thickness and density. Pacing Clin. Electrophysiol. **36**(1), 55–62 (2013). doi:10.1111/pace.12028

8. Inoue, J., Baxter, J.S.H., Drangova, M.: Left atrial wall segmentation from CT for radiofrequency catheter ablation planning. In: Oyarzun Laura, C., Shekhar, R., Wesarg, S., González Ballester, M.Á., Drechsler, K., Sato, Y., Erdt, M., Linguraru, M.G. (eds.) CLIP 2015. LNCS, vol. 9401, pp. 71–78. Springer, Heidelberg (2016). doi:10.1007/978-3-319-31808-0_9

9. Inoue, J., Skanes, A.C., White, J.A., Rajchl, M., Drangova, M.: Patient-specific left atrial wall-thickness measurement and visualization for radiofrequency ablation. In: SPIE Medical Imaging, vol. 9036, id. 90361N (2014). doi:10.1117/12.2043630

10. STACOM Left Atrial Wall Thickness Challenge

11. Cochet, H., Dubois, R., Sacher, F., Derval, N., Sermesant, M., Hocini, M., Montaudon, M., Haïssaguerre, M., Laurent, F., Jaïs, P.: Cardiac arrythmias: multimodal assessment integrating body surface ECG mapping into cardiac imaging. Radiology **271**(1), 239–247 (2013). doi:10.1148/radiol.13131331

12. Jean, S.: Image Analysis and Mathematical Morphology. Academic Press Inc., Orlando (1983)

13. Pei, S.-C., Lai, C.-L., Shih, F.Y.: An efficient class of alternating sequential filters in morphology. Graph. Models Image Process. **59**(2), 109–116 (1997). doi:10.1006/gmip.1996.0416

14. Caselles, V., Kimmel, R., Sapiro, G.: Geodesic active contours. Int. J. Comput. Vis. **22**(1), 61–79 (1997). doi:10.1023/A:1007979827043

15. Huda, W.: Review of Radiologic Physics. Lippincott Williams and Wilkins, Philadelphia (2010)

16. Varela, M., Kolbitsch, C., Theron, A., Morgan, R., Henningsson, M., Schaeffter, T., Aslanidi, O.: 3D high-resolution atrial wall thickness maps using blackblood PSIR. J. Cardiovasc. Magn. Reson. **17**(Suppl 1), 239 (2015). doi:10.1186/1532-429X-17-S1-P239

Automatic Left Atrial Wall Segmentation from Contrast-Enhanced CT Angiography Images

Qian Tao$^{(\boxtimes)}$, Rahil Shahzad, Floris F. Berendsen, and Rob J. van der Geest

Division of Image Processing (LKEB), Department of Radiology,
Leiden University Medical Center, Leiden, The Netherlands
q.tao@lumc.nl

Abstract. Assessment of the left atrial (LA) wall can provide valuable information for treatment of atrial fibrillation (AF) patients. In this work, we propose a fully automatic workflow to segment the atrial wall from contrast-enhanced CT angiography (CTA). The workflow consists of 3 steps: (1) global segmentation of LA by multi-atlas image registration approach, (2) selected enhancement of the atrial wall by nonlinear intensity transformation, (3) segmentation of the inner and outer boundary of atrial wall by level-set approach.

Keywords: CTA · Atrial wall segmentation · Multi-atlas · Level-set

1 Introduction

Atrial fibrillation (AF) is the most common cardiac electrophysiological disorder worldwide [5]. Previous studies have shown that tissue characteristics of the left atrium (LA) wall can provide valuable information for determining the appropriate strategy of catheter ablation for AF patients [3]. However, it remains difficult to assess the atrial wall with non-invasive imaging techniques, as visualizing the atrial wall demands both high resolution and high soft tissue contrast. In clinical practice, contrast-enhanced CT angiography (CTA) is frequently used to examine the LA geometry. CTA delineates the blood pool with high contrast at sub-millimetre resolution, but has poor soft tissue contrast for visualizing the atrial wall. To automatically segment the atrial wall from CTA is challenging in at least two ways: firstly, for initialization of the atrial wall segmentation, the LA needs to be segmented in the first place, which itself has a complex geometry with variable pulmonary veins (PV) location; secondly, the contrast between the atrial wall and surroundings is typically very poor, and can hardly be appreciated by eye, especially when the layer of atrial wall spans only a few voxels.

In this work, we propose a fully automated left atrial wall segmentation workflow which combines three major parts: (1) automatic LA blood pool segmentation; (2) atrial wall enhancement; and (3) atrial wall segmentation.

© Springer International Publishing AG 2017
T. Mansi et al. (Eds.): STACOM 2016, LNCS 10124, pp. 220–227, 2017.
DOI: 10.1007/978-3-319-52718-5_24

2   Data and Method

2.1   CTA Data

Ten datasets were available from the *MICCAI 2016 Left Atrial Wall Thickness Challenge*. For each subject, coronary CTA was performed on a Philips 256 iCT scanner. All patients were injected with an intravenous contrast agent. The scans were ECG-gated and image acquisition was performed in a single breath hold. The images were reconstructed to a 0.8 to 1 mm slice thickness, with a 0.4 mm slice increment and a 250 mm field of view. The image matrix was kept at 512 × 512 matrix, constructed with a sharp reconstruction kernel. Figure 1 shows 2 example CTA image from the dataset.

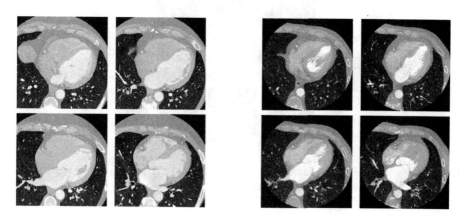

Fig. 1. Two examples of the CTA database from MICCAI 2016 Left Atrial Wall Thickness Challenge.

2.2   Global LA Segmentation

A multi-atlas segmentation approach was used to derive an initial global segmentation of the LA and PV's connected to it. We used the atlases from our magnetic resonance angiography (MRA) study [6], in which 10 MRA dataset were selected based on two criteria: (1) good image quality, (2) representative of the LA and PV morphology. An experienced observer carefully annotated the LA and PVs in each of the 10 dataset.

The rationale of the multi-atlas segmentation method is illustrated by Fig. 2: first each of the 10 atlases was registered to the given image, then the 10 known segmentations were propagated to the given image so that each voxel has 10 votes; finally the majority-vote was obtained to provide the labeling of the LA and PV regions in the given image. For each atlas, rigid registration was first applied to roughly align the atlas to the given image, followed by a non-rigid registration with B-spline to match them in a flexible and refined manner. Normalized mutual information was used as the optimization criterion, and adaptive

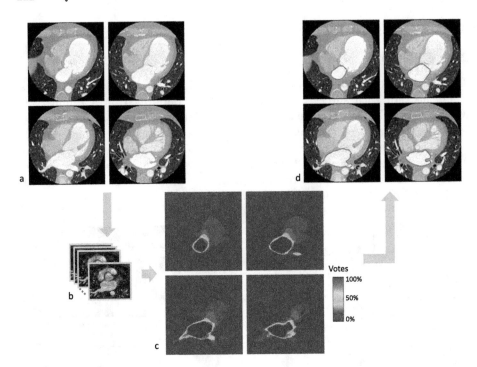

Fig. 2. Diagram of multi-atlas registration: a. Original CTA image to be segmented, b. Multiple atlases with known segmentation, c. Votes (in percentage) from different atlases after registration, d. Segmentation results by majority vote.

stochastic gradient descent method was used as the optimization routine [2]. For non-rigid registration we set the B-spline grid to the empirical value of 30 mm, which is sufficiently small to accommodate the inter-subject variability, while large enough to prevent unrealistic deformation.

2.3 Atrial Wall Enhancement

The limited soft tissue contrast in CTA makes it difficult to visually discern the thin atrial wall, see Fig. 1. We propose to first enhance the object, i.e., the atrial wall, using prior knowledge of the tissue Hounsfield unit (HU).

The atrial wall that we intend to segment borders the LA blood pool (inner surface) and epicardial fat (outer surface). In literature, it is documented that the HU for myocardial tissue with enhancement ranges between 100 to 300, while epicardial fat has a HU range of −100 to −50 [1]. Considering the partial volume effect between the high-HU contrast-enhanced blood, thin atrial wall, and low-HU fat, we set the dynamic range to [0 400] as the region of interest for atrial wall search. Figure 3b shows the adjusted CTA image excluding fat around the LA.

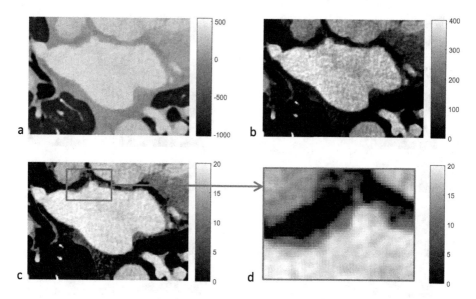

Fig. 3. a. The original CTA image with high intensity range. b. The CTA image within range [0 400], with fat tissue removed. c. The CTA image with nonlinear operation to reduce the dynamic range. d. Zoomed-in part in c.

As the contrast-enhanced blood pool has high brightness, the fine structure of the atrial wall is often "overshadowed". We subsequently apply a nonlinear transform to suppress the bright signals to enhance the atrial wall within the [0 400] range. In principle, any nonlinear transformation that suppresses large signals more than small signals, such as logarithm, square root, can be used for atrial wall enhancement. Figure 3c shows the resulting image with square root operation (from [0 400] to [0 20]), and the zoomed-in version of d illustrates a thin layer of atrial wall, which is better visible than in Fig. 3a or b.

2.4   Dual Atrial Wall Segmentation

The global LA segmentation by the multi-atlas method is robust and reliable, but it can be relatively inaccurate at border regions where the agreement from atlases reduces, see Fig. 2c. Consequently, a few voxels displacement may cause the thin atrial wall being missed. In this step, we use a level-set approach [4] to obtain the inner and outer atrial surface in a three-dimensional manner.

A level set function Φ is defined in three-dimensional space, which has positive values inside and negative values outside the surface, which is denoted by $\Phi(x, y, z) = 0$. The dynamics to evolve the three-dimensional surface can be imposed in its normal direction, by image forces derived from the original CTA image, as expressed by

$$\Phi_t + F|\nabla\Phi| = 0 \tag{1}$$

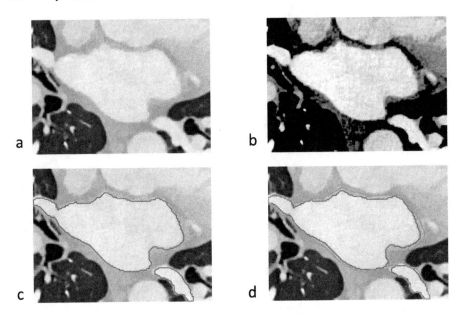

Fig. 4. a. The original CTA image. b. The enhance image. c. Inner contour overlaid by the first level set operation. d. Outer contour overlaid by the second level set operation.

where $\Phi_t = \frac{\partial \Phi}{\partial t}$ describes the evolving of Φ, and in this work, the image force F is defined as a combination of image gradient and region information to evolve the implicit surface, as described in [7].

A unique property of the level-set method approach is that it does not have prior assumptions on the morphology and can thus deal with complex shapes like the LA plus PVs. Starting from the multi-atlas segmentation, we applied a first level set to grow the initial segmentation to the inner surface of LA, see Fig. 4c. Then we applied a second level set using the inner surface as the initialization, and grow it to the outer boundary as shown in Fig. 4d. The second level set was evolved based on image gradient from the enhanced image described in Sect. 2.3. Meanwhile, we imposed prior knowledge, i.e. the atrial wall thickness is in the range of 1–4 mm, by limiting the level-set growth. We have applied two constraints: first, the level-set to detect the outer wall was confined with a region of 4 mm thickness from the inner wall; second, the number of iterations was limited to $4/s$, where s is the in-plane resolution of the CTA image. Figure 5 shows two examples of the automatic atrial wall segmentation results in 2D.

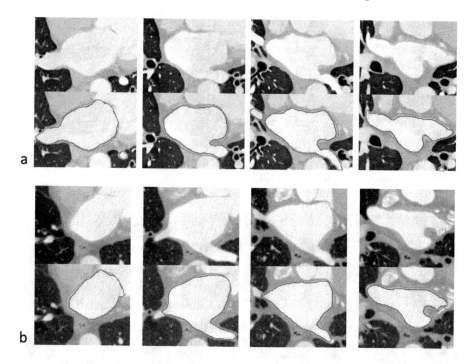

Fig. 5. Two examples of the automatic atrial segmentation result.

3 Results

3.1 Segmentation Results

In total 3 dataset, namely CT2, CT3, and CT5, were manually segmented. We compared our automatic segmentation results to the manual segmentation. Figure 6 shows the comparison between manual and automatic segmentation in 3D, while Fig. 7 shows the comparison in 2D slices. The Dice indice were computed as 0.51, 0.43, and 0.43 for the three cases, respectively. It is observed that part of the atrial wall in manual segmentation is missing, possibly due to the difficulty to discern the signal intensity difference at local areas, while in our automatic method the atrial wall is always continuous.

3.2 Limitations

The accuracy of atrial wall segmentation is dependent on the CTA quality. A high resolution in the order of half a millimetre is necessary to differentiate the LA wall voxels, and meanwhile motion artefacts should be minimal which would otherwise cause a false low-intensity rim mistaken as the atrial wall.

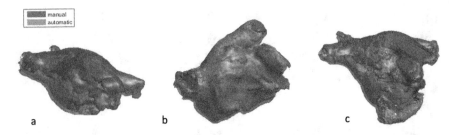

Fig. 6. Comparison of 3D shape between the manual and automatic segmentation in 3 available cases: a. CT2, b. CT3, c. CT5.

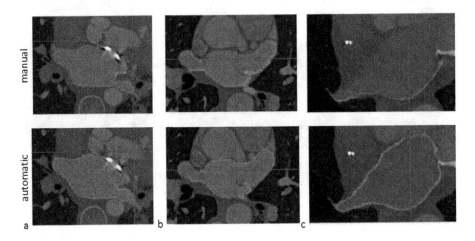

Fig. 7. Comparison of 2D annotation between the manual and automatic segmentation in 3 available cases: a. CT2, b. CT3, c. CT5. The upper panel is the manual segmentation, and the lower panel is the automatic segmentation.

4   Conclusion

We have developed a fully automatic workflow to segment the atrial wall from CTA images consisting of three steps, LA blood pool segmentation, LA wall enhancement, and LA wall segmentation. The method allows objective evaluation of the atrial wall, the underlying substrate of arrhythmias originating from atrium, potentially leading to improved interventional strategy for the large AF population.

Acknowledgement. The authors gratefully acknowledge the support from the Dutch Technology Foundation, with grant number OTP12899.

References

1. De Vos, W., Casselman, J., Swennen, G.: Cone-beam computerized tomography imaging of the oral and maxillofacial region: a systematic review of the literature. Int. J. Oral Maxillofac. Surg. **38**, 609–625 (2009)
2. Klein, S., Staring, M., Murphy, K., Viergever, M., Pluim, J.: Elastix: a toolbox for intensity-based medical image registration. IEEE Trans. Med. Imaging **29**, 196–205 (2010)
3. Marrouche, N., Wilber, D., Hindricks, G., Jais, P., Akoum, N., Marchlinski, F., Kholmovski, E., Burgon, N., Hu, N., Mont, L., Deneke, T., Duytschaever, M., Neumann, T., Mansour, M., Mahnkopf, C., Herweg, B., Daoud, E., Wissner, E., Bansmann, P., Brachmann, J.: Association of atrial tissue fibrosis identified by delayed enhancement MRI and atrial fibrillation catheter ablation: the DECAAF study. JAMA **11**, 85–92 (2014)
4. Osher, S., Sethian, J.: Fronts propagating with curvature dependent speed: algorithms based on Hamilton-Jacobi formulations. J. Comput. Phys. **28**, 907–922 (1988)
5. Prystowsky, E., Benson, D.J., Fuster, V., Hart, R., Kay, G., Myerburg, R., Naccarelli, G., Wyse, D.: Management of patients with atrial fibrillation. A statement for healthcare professionals. From the subcommittee on electrocardiography and electrophysiology, American heart association. Circulation **93**, 1262–1277 (1996)
6. Tao, Q., Ipek, E., Shahzad, R., Berendsen, F., Nazarian, S., van der Geest, R.: Fully automatic segmentation of left atrium and pulmonary veins in late gadolinium-enhanced MRI: towards objective atrial scar assessment. J. Magn. Reson. Imaging **44**(2), 346–354 (2016)
7. Zhang, Y., Matuszewski, B.J., Shark, L.K., Moore, C.J.: Medical image segmentation using new hybrid level-set method. In: Proceedings of the 2008 Fifth International Conference BioMedical Visualization: Information Visualization in Medical and Biomedical Informatics. MEDIVIS 2008, pp. 71–76. IEEE Computer Society, Washington, DC (2008)

Author Index

Printed in the United States
By Bookmasters